Herpes Simplex

Though medically minor and very common, herpes simplex is a condition which is capable of causing considerable distress, for psychological and social as much as physical reasons. *Herpes Simplex* contrasts the image of the condition presented in the media with the medical and epidemiological evidence, and discusses ways in which the distress associated with the condition can be alleviated. The first part of the book examines the impact of diagnosis and then explains the roles of accurate information and empathic support, medical treatment and support groups in learning to live with recurrent symptoms. Other chapters use the experiences of people with the condition in different parts of their bodies to illustrate how the meaning of herpes simplex and response to the symptoms alters in association with life changes. The final chapters review psychosocial research, discuss the importance of the Herpes Viruses Association in acquiring a store of knowledge about people's experiences, and highlight the significance of herpes simplex as a public health problem.

Herpes Simplex demonstrates the importance of a biopsychosocial approach. It will be invaluable to doctors, nurses and other health professionals, as well as to people troubled by the condition.

T. Natasha Posner is Lecturer in Medical Sociology at the University of Queensland, Australia.

The Experience of Illness

Series Editors: Ray Fitzpatrick and Stanton Newman

Herpes Simplex

T. Natasha Posner

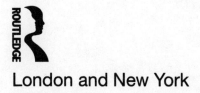

London and New York

First published 1998 by Routledge
11 New Fetter Lane, London EC4P 4EE

Simultaneously published in the USA and Canada
by Routledge
29 West 35th Street, New York, NY 10001

© 1998 T. Natasha Posner

Typeset in Times by Routledge
Printed and bound in Great Britain by Page Brothers (Norwich) Ltd

British Library Cataloguing in Publication Data
A catalogue record for this book is available from the British Library

Library of Congress Cataloging in Publication Data
Posner, T. Natasha, 1942–
Herpes simplex /T. Natasha Posner.
p. cm. – (The Experience of illness)
Includes bibliographical references and index.
1. Herpes simplex – Social aspects. 2. Herpes simplex – Psychological
aspects. I. Title. II. Series.
RC147.H6P67   1988
362.1'969518–dc21   97-17152
                                                              CIP

ISBN 0–415–10744–X

Contents

Editors' preface

The monographs in this series illustrate a fundamental theme. Physical illness needs to be understood at two quite different levels of reality. At one level the body is challenged by threats to biological processes. At another level illnesses have personal and social significance that cannot be reduced to biology. Natasha Posner's account of herpes simplex perfectly illustrates this twin dynamic. In many cases, infection with the herpes simplex virus is a mild event with few serious consequences for the body. However, to the individual who experiences infection, the diagnosis may be extremely distressing. How the virus can have these two very different kinds of impact, at the biological and psychosocial levels, is described by Natasha Posner with a persuasive and careful analysis of her materials and elegant narrative.

The book is based on a rich range of resources. She draws on up-to-date explanantions of herpes simplex from the medical literature. At the same time she has extensively examined the popular media's treatment of the subject. The media have created an image of a pervasive and threatening infection. It is often treated in moralistic terms as a by-product of the sexual revolution. Natasha Posner also sought the accounts of the lives of individuals who had experienced symptoms of the virus. They report shock, devastation and anger at the time of diagnosis. For some symptoms will be recurrent and individuals have to adjust to a chronic problem. Accurate information and support from others, particularly others with experience of the condition seems often to be far more beneficial than the response from the medical profession.

By challenging the negative cultural meanings of this virus Natasha Posner provides fundamental guidance towards more appropriate care for herpes simplex.

Ray Fitzpatrick, 1997

Author's preface

Much has been written about herpes simplex, both in the medical literature and in the popular press, often with a focus on rare medical complications of infection or worst case scenarios. This has left most of the usual experience of the condition out of the picture, since it was of little concern as a medical problem and of little interest as a story.

The challenge of this book has been to produce a more balanced presentation, and to accurately portray symptom recurrences as a chronic condition embedded in the complex interrelations of mind, body and social context. To try to do this, the book has drawn on a variety of data sources and a wide range of written material including newspaper and magazine articles, pamphlets and academic journal papers in the medical, epidemiological and psychosocial literature. It has been immensely enriched by all those people who have shared their experiences of herpes simplex on survey questionnaires, in interviews, or by writing about them. They have contributed to a growth in our understanding of the nature and impact of this condition and the different ways in which people respond to and live with herpes simplex. I am indebted to them for material presented in this book.

I would particularly like to acknowledge all that I have learnt during my association over a decade with the Herpes Association (now Herpes Viruses Association) in London, and from Mike Wolfe and Marian Nicholson especially. I first made contact with the association when I was carrying on research among self-help organisations in the health field, and was impressed by the association's role in supporting individuals, providing comprehensive information and representing people troubled by herpes simplex.

I want to thank my friends and colleagues in England and

Queensland who have borne my enthusiasms and frustrations during the writing process with equanimity. I have been very grateful for Ray Fitzpatrick's encouragement and editorial wisdom. I would also like to thank Jenny Berzins, Fred de Looze and Mandy Hudson from the Department of Social and Preventive Medicine at the University of Queensland for their help with typing the final version of the manuscript.

I am also grateful to the following: Sage Publications for permission to reproduce material from J. M. Swanson and W. C. Chenitz (1993) 'Regaining a valued self: the process of adaptation to living with genital herpes' *Qualitative Health Research* 3(3): 270–97; Baywood Publishing Co. for permission to reproduce material from David Longo and Kent Koehn (1993) 'Psychosocial factors and recurrent genital herpes: a review of prediction and psychiatric treatment studies' *International Journal of Psychiatry in Medicine* 23(2): 99–117; JAI Press for permission to reproduce material from Kathy Charmaz (1987) 'Struggling for self: identity levels of the chronically ill' *Research in the Sociology of Health Care* 6: 283–321; Cambridge University Press for permission to reproduce material from Nancy Waxler (1981) 'Learning to be a leper: a case study in the social construction of illness' in E. Mishler *et al.* (eds) *Social Contexts of Health, Illness and Patient Care*; Tavistock for permission to reproduce material from G. Scambler (1984) 'Perceiving and coping with stigmatizing illness' in R. Fitzpatrick *et al.* (eds) *The Experience of Illness*.

The book has been written in the hope that it may contribute in some way to our living more easily with this common condition which has coexisted so successfully with us.

Chapter 1

Introduction
The cultural, epidemiological and biomedical context

This book is not about a disease confined to a small minority of people but about a condition that most of the population have acquired, but do not suffer. Herpes simplex is a very common infection, but it rarely causes illness. Where it does cause suffering, the distress comes as much, if not more, from the image of the condition as from the physical symptoms. The psychosocial elements in the experience of herpes simplex are crucial. These elements are shaped by the personal and social context in which the condition is experienced.

Very different views of the condition exist. The medical profession's general view of herpes simplex is that it is not a significant medical problem except on very rare occasions, or when a patient is immunocompromised. Dr Adrian Mindel, an acknowledged expert on herpes simplex infection (and at that time GUM consultant at London's Middlesex Hospital), told the *Independent* (21 July 1987):

> For the majority of people herpes is a minor viral complaint; it is nothing more than an occasional nuisance.

Urologist Peter Gross spoke admiringly to *Time* magazine (2 August 1982) about the ability of herpes viruses to secrete themselves in the human bodily system:

> By any measure, herpes is an extraordinary bug ... If you were doing a science fiction movie, you couldn't invent something better than herpes.

Professor Mike Adler, quoted in the *Daily Express* (7 February 1983) said:

> The disease is definitely sexually transmitted and so far there is

no cure. But we need to see it for what it is, a minor non-life threatening complaint.

Levenson and co-workers (1987) wrote that:

Genital herpes simplex infection is a major personal and public health problem affecting millions of patients.

Thus, among specialists, herpes simplex is 'a minor viral complaint', 'an extraordinary bug', a sexually-transmitted disease, and 'a major . . . public health problem' depending on which aspect of the condition is the focus of attention.

For one organisation representing people troubled by the condition, it is a 'natural part' of human life and one which has been with us for a long time:

Herpes simplex itself is a natural part and fact of life – one we can live in harmony with if we can accept it in its true perspective.

(Herpes Association 1993a: 10)

The Herpes simplex virus has probably evolved and developed with humans since the dawn of time. It was certainly well known to the ancient Greeks from whom the virus acquired its name. The virus is found universally, knows no boundaries of class, creed or race and will infect any part of the body where it can gain access. Herpes simplex is a parasitic virus and is the most successful of all the herpes viruses, successful in that it has adapted itself so well to us, the hosts. At some time in their life almost everyone comes into contact with the virus and are infected – with or without symptoms.

(ibid.: 9)

In the 1980s, herpes simplex received intense attention from the popular media. This both increased awareness of the condition, and created a very negative popular image of it. Herpes simplex became a problem in a way it had not been before. The nature of this problem needs to be considered against the background of its cultural, epidemiological and biomedical contexts.

THE CULTURAL CONTEXT

A *BMJ* editorial on 4 June 1983 was headlined 'Genital herpes: hype or hope?' and began:

Genital herpes has received enormous attention by the media during the past year, and many of the articles have been sensational, inaccurate and of little help to patients.

(Adler and Mindel 1983)

There was certainly little hope in the hype which presented the condition in the worst possible light, distorting the facts and exaggerating the significance of ill effects – in the process creating a monster out of a common and minor condition which had quietly co-existed with humans for a very long time. The meanings heaped on this condition were enough to take it to the top of the league of feared sexually transmitted infections, and in themselves, irrespective of the nature of any physical manifestations, to cause very significant psychosocial and psychosexual morbidity.

The condition was presented as sweeping through the ranks of the sexually active with an incidence reaching epidemic proportions.

Today this viral infection has . . . established itself as an uncontrollable epidemic.

(*Cosmopolitan*, July 1982)

Herpes has emerged from relative obscurity and exploded into a full-fledged epidemic.

(*Time*, 2 August 1982)

A new and as yet incurable disease, spread through sex contact has reached epidemic proportions in parts of the Western world.

(*Daily Mail*, 28 July 1982)

The *Daily Mail* article quoted above was in the 'Femail' section and headlined 'Nature's new threat to women' and, to emphasise the pervasiveness of the threat, suggested that you may be an ordinary woman in a typical role, but you only have to step outside the bounds of sexual propriety once to join the ranks of 'victims':

Nor is the problem confined as is commonly supposed to women who make a habit of 'sleeping around'. Herpes is now so widespread that victims are often housewives, teachers and secretaries who may have been guilty of only one act of sexual indiscretion.

Joanna Day in the *Observer* (5 December 1982) attempting to put the claims into perspective, wrote:

Statistics for England and Wales, meanwhile, show that *if* there is an epidemic on this side of the Atlantic, it is one of fear rather than fact.

Fear of the infection would certainly have been encouraged by the media presentations of its nature: 'Sexually transmitted herpes – highly contagious, incurable and unpredictably recurrent' (*Observer*, 2 May 1982); 'Herpes: the New Sexual Leprosy' (*Time*, 28 July 1980). The condition was presented as not only incurable, but having serious medical and psychosexual sequelae.

For a self-limiting condition which bodily defences normally deal with very adequately without medical intervention so that it is 'cured' every time it occurs, 'incurable' is clearly an emotionally loaded word. Many people who are infected with HSV do not appear to have recurrences and are unaware of symptoms. The infection produces antibodies while the virus lies dormant in the body, as do many others, for instance, varicella (chicken pox) which may in later life return to symptomatic mode as herpes zoster (shingles). Though HSV symptoms can now be suppressed by treatment with acyclovir, the antiviral drug was only just being introduced at this time. The unpredictable recurrence of symptom episodes is undoubtedly a difficult aspect of living with the condition, and has resulted in the attribution of negative anthropomorphic characteristics to the activity of the virus, and suggestions that it has 'a mind of its own' (*Time*, 2 August 1982) with which it chooses to play havoc with its victims' lives, leaving them at its mercy. A sufferer quoted in *Cosmopolitan* (July 1982) said:

I felt like a victim. It's frustrating to be subject to a little tiny virus that messes things up.

Writing about the obscurity of the mechanisms which provoke re-emergence, Collee (1994) suggested that:

at times the virus seems almost wilfully malicious . . . like having a tedious relation who unerringly chooses the most inappropriate moments to come and stay.

One of the scare stories which accompanied most articles about herpes in the early eighties related to the risk of cervical cancer, eg.:

There is a strong suggestion of high risk of cervical cancer in women who have had herpes, especially HSV-2 of the cervix. They are recommended to have six-monthly smear tests.

(*Spare Rib* 1980)

Herpes has now been associated in many studies with another, extremely serious disease – cancer of the cervix . . . and it may well turn out to be the cause of it.

(Sunday Times, 5 December 1982)

In women, recurrent attacks are thought to increase the risk of cervical cancer between five and eightfold.

(Observer, 2 May 1982)

Herpes has been linked to cancer of the cervix, which afflicts an estimated 16,000 US women in its serious form and contributes to 7,400 deaths a year.

(Time, 28 July 1980)

A most dramatic presentation of this postulated link was spelt out in *Cosmopolitan* (January 1984) in which an article suggested that there was 'evidence that . . . HSV-2 may be a trigger for cervical cancer', and that women with cervical cancer or pre-cancerous conditions of the cervix had been found to have 'high levels of anti-bodies to genital herpes in their blood and cervical mucus'.

Laboratory tests have shown that if cells in a culture are exposed to the HSV-2 virus and then injected into hamsters, the animals develop tumours. While most viruses just kill the cell, the HSV-2 virus can turn the cell itself into a killer. Cells can become cancerous, yet the mechanism is so subtle that no trace of the deadly intruder is left behind – with no virus genetic material remaining to positively incriminate it. The herpes virus has the special ability to deliver a hit and run attack.

The negativity and metaphor of the language of this extract is typical of articles about herpes simplex around this time. The finding of a correlation between abnormal cervical cells and anti-bodies to HSV-2 was misinterpreted as a causal connection. In this case, the wrong virus was being implicated as a causal factor, and it was later found that certain versions of Human Papilloma Virus (HPV) were significant in the aetiology of cervical cancer and its precursors.

The *Cosmopolitan* article (January 1984) mentioned above contained several of the other scary warnings which were often reproduced in the media. One of these was the idea of self-inoculation, transfer-ence of the condition from one part of the body to another. The suggestion was that infection from the 'cold sore' version of the virus (HSV-1) could be transferred from the face to the person's own genitals: 'It's all too easy for this to happen during sleep through simple scratching'. The article went on to warn against the risk of using 'strange or unclean towels' as:

> towels can spread herpes, too, as the organism can survive on them for some time to provide a source of infection for anyone else using the same towel.

If the risk of transference of herpetic infection by self-inoculation or from towels was at all likely, one would expect many more instances of symptoms occurring on the hands or various other parts of the body than there are.

Another, highly emotive scare story which has been almost invariably mentioned in the media coverage of genital herpes simplex, relates to the neonatal risk of mothers passing on the condition to their babies. Again the facts were distorted and presented in the worst light:

> There is no doubt that herpes can be passed on to newborn babies if mothers have an active infection at the time of delivery. Each year several hundred babies are born with herpes simplex; more than half die, and survivors often suffer permanent neurological damage.
>
> (*Time*, 28 July 1980)

> In a British study of 302 babies born with herpes, 60% died; only 22% had no ill-effects . . . women who plan to have children face particularly frightening risks . . . babies can pick up the virus in the birth canal if the mother is suffering an outbreak at the time of delivery . . . The virus quickly spreads through the infants' bodies, killing more than half of them and leaving most of the survivors permanently brain-damaged.
>
> (*Cosmopolitan*, July 1982)

> A child who is delivered vaginally while the mother has an active attack of HSV-2 is likely to catch the virus through its eyes, skin or mouth. Two thirds of babies infected in this way die, and most who survive suffer severe damage to their brain or eyes.
>
> (*Spare Rib* 1980)

A cursory look at the prevalence of HSV-2 infection among adults, alongside the statistics for neonatal herpes simplex infection, would have raised doubts about the nature of the risk because of the large number of babies being born vaginally to women with HSV-2 antibodies who did not suffer herpetic symptoms (see discussion below). The possible psychological and emotional sequelae of the condition were presented in equally lurid tones as if they were inevitable accompaniments. 'Not only is the disease dangerous physically – it also causes a great deal of psychological distress' *Cosmopolitan* (July 1982) suggested, before spelling out the nature of this suffering. Among the millions of Americans 'believed to suffer from herpes':

> Virtually all of them . . . must endure an emotional crisis so distinct in its assault on their sense of worth that psychologists speak of a 'herpes syndrome'. Herpes victims find themselves suddenly beset by new vulnerabilities and moral dilemmas. They feel tainted, fearful that no one will ever want to love them.

The article continued in the same tones, spelling out the author's interpretation of the 'herpes syndrome' postulated by Luby and Gillespie (1981): 'a pattern of anguish and isolation that may play havoc with a person's self-image and social life for years while he [*sic*] comes to terms with his disease'. And then there are the psychosexual consequences:

> For single people, herpes may shatter relationships or render a formerly fulfilling social life erratic and frustrating. For couples who are married or living together, herpes may strain the relationship to breaking point.

Doyle in the *Observer* (2 May 1982) wrote that much publicity had been given in the USA to 'the devastating emotional and psychological anguish of possessing an incurable sexually transmitted disease', suggesting that 'with herpes . . . the blow to a satisfactory sex life and to sexual self-esteem may be shattering'. An article in *Time* (28 July 1980) with the heading 'Herpes: The New Sexual Leprosy. "Viruses of love" infect millions with disease and despair' suggested that 'most will suffer shame, guilt and even depression, and a few will become suicidal', and quoted an informant who said:

> I regard myself as a carrier of an invisible, incurable disease. I have a guilt trip that won't quit.

Ten years later, the 'psychological effects' of the condition were still being written about as if they were a necessary accompaniment of the physical symptoms:

The symbolic meaning of herpes and its effects on self-esteem and body image have the greatest destructive impact, and sufferers move through a sequence of adaptational responses remarkably similar to those described for cancer.

(Beardsley 1993)

This sentence is almost a word for word repetition of part of the abstract of the paper by Luby and Klinge (1985) which reported findings of a small survey of support group members and clinic patients in New York. This author, writing for a nursing audience, then listed, unquestioned, supposed psychosocial responses to HSV infection as:

depression (50 per cent), avoidance of intimate relationships (53 per cent), impotence and reduced libido (35 per cent), reduced work performance (40 per cent), cessation of all sexual activity (10 per cent).

(Beardsley 1993)

The article was entitled 'Education to undermine a taboo', but the repetition of early commentaries on biased samples at the height of the media hype in the USA, as if they were facts about the condition, could only serve to feed the taboo.

By the early 1990s, some of the other misconceptions, for instance about modes of transmission, were being corrected. An article in *Family Circle*'s 'health fact file' (April 1993) stated:

It is possible to catch genital herpes by having oral sex with someone who has a cold sore. However, there is no evidence to suggest that the virus can be transferred from your face to your genital area by touch, except during your very first attack.

Marie Claire (August 1993, UK edition) reassured that herpes simplex is 'not transmitted by sharing cups, towels, toilet seats, bath water or swimming pools' and that 'despite much misinformation in the 1980s, cervical cancer is not causally related to HSV'. Memuna Forna in the *Guardian* (30 May 1991) attempted to set the record straight in relation to the risk of pregnant women passing the infection to their babies:

The virus has been associated with foetal defects, but many of the scare stories have now been disproved. There are in fact only two areas of risk: if a woman gets HSV during the early stages of pregnancy, she may miscarry and if a sore is present just prior to birth.

Under the headline 'What happened to the herpes plague?', Frances Hubbard in the *Daily Express* (17 October 1990) wrote of the commonness and relative harmlessness of the condition:

> By middle-age, 90 per cent of us have antibodies to the virus in our blood. It is only the unlucky few who get those dreaded blisters . . .
>
> Most live happily with it without suffering a single symptom . . . The truth is that herpes has existed for at least 2000 years without posing any serious threat to humanity.

Early in the decade of the eighties, this minor self-limiting infection was attributed a significant societal role in bringing about a fundamental change in sexual mores. Referred to as 'this perplexing side-effect of the sexual revolution' (*Observer*, 2 May 1982), and 'a new, alarming by-product of the sexual revolution' (*Cosmopolitan*, July 1982), it was suggested that 'The herpes counterrevolution may be ushering a reluctant, grudging chastity back into fashion' (*Time*, 2 August 1982). 'Does this contagious, recurrent disease spell the end of the permissive society?' the *Reader's Digest* asked in 1983. If there were deep-seated changes in attitudes towards sexual relations at this time, they were triggered by fears and anxieties associated with and symbolised by HSV, rather than any inherent characteristic of the condition itself, harboured unknowingly and without distress by the majority of the population.

An indication of the sociocultural significance of herpes simplex can be gained from the analysis of its dramatic role in at least two films from the USA shown on television. How many other STDs have been given such a key part in popular dramas? Chlamydia has a promising-sounding name, and has indeed been featured in *Neighbours*, and syphilis has certainly been in the background of several stories, but neither had a crucially important role in the unfolding of the drama itself. *Intimate Agony*, shown on BBC TV Channel 4 in 1985, revolves around the implications of the spread of HSV amongst the residents of an American offshore island resort. A young woman declares 'My life is over' when she learns her diagnosis from a clinic doctor. When she tells her best friend, the friend recoils from her in horror and refuses even to touch an item of her clothing. A husband passes the virus to his pregnant wife who gives birth prematurely to a brain-damaged baby who dies. A flirtatious tennis coach has his self-confidence destroyed and begins to avoid sexual encounters after contracting the infection.

Acyclovir was mentioned as a treatment early in the film, and one of the doctors involved was sympathetic and supportive; the ending was focused on the meeting of a self-help group, but overall the film dwelt on the most negative implications of HSV and was likely to have perpetuated existing myths. As a reviewer in the HA newsletter *Sphere* wrote:

> the film's real impact is on an emotional level and the viewer is left with images of broken relationships, dead babies and people who are emotionally crippled by shame, fear and guilt.
>
> (*Sphere* 1985 (2): 2)

In August 1993 a two-part drama by Scott Turow with the title *The Burden of Proof* was shown on BBC TV Channel 1. The film is about a defence lawyer's attempt to unravel the mystery of his wife's suicide with which the film begins. One of the secrets he uncovers is that his wife had recurring genital symptoms of HSV, and that when they 'got bad' she had said 'I'm really not sure I can carry on' and had talked of suicide. The condition was referred to in the film as 'a disease', 'an illness', 'the mortal hazards of an STD' and 'repulsive'. The wife was reported as saying that she was being treated for something 'unmentionable'. Acyclovir, however, was mentioned. The condition was thus presented in the film in a highly stigmatised way and as being implicated, along with other factors, in the wife's suicide.

THE EPIDEMIOLOGICAL CONTEXT

The epidemiological evidence relating to HSV has been largely based on Genitourinary Medicine (GUM) and Sexually Transmitted Disease (STD) clinic reports and laboratory documentation. As much HSV infection will result in only mild symptoms, or none at all, so that the individuals involved will not seek medical help, the majority of infections will not be counted from clinic and laboratory reports. We do not have an accurate picture of the prevalence of the two types of HSV fifteen or more years ago as accurate serotyping was not possible. Such evidence as there is suggests that HSV infection was endemic. In recent years accurate serotyping has been possible, and surveys have been carried out in certain populations to assess the prevalence of HSV-1 and HSV-2 infection. However, 'there are no true population-based data' and there is a case for 'national population-based surveys of HSV-2 and HPV morbidity' (Donovan and Mindel 1995). It appears that genital infection has increased, but it remains difficult to know to what extent this is due to changed sexual practices in relation to oral sex (between 20 per cent and 60 per cent of primary genital HSV infections in Britain being due to HSV-1 (Patel, Cowan and Barton 1997)), or to increased attendance at clinics, or to a genuine spread of HSV-2 infection, or to increased ability to distinguish HSV-1 from HSV-2.

An analysis published in 1990 by the World Health Organization estimated that worldwide there were 250 million sexually transmitted infections annually, of which 120 million were trichomoniasis, 50 million were chlamydia, 30 million were genital warts, and 20 million genital herpes (WHO 1990). An editorial in the *BMJ* in 1983 (Adler and Mindel 1983) estimated that of half a million cases of sexually transmitted disease seen annually in clinics in Britain, only 12,000 were genital herpes (2 per cent), however, there had been an apparent increase in the previous five years of 60 per cent.

The Office of Population Censuses and Surveys (OPCS) table of 'Identifications of viruses, chlamydias, rickettsias and mycoplasmas' (Table 13 Series MB2 No.7, England and Wales) shows herpes simplex cases increasing from 5,044 to 7,404 in 1980; chlamydia A from 1,100 to 3,292. By 1986, identifications of herpes simplex had more than doubled and chlamydia A had increased sevenfold, to 16,995 and 29,599 respectively. Listing of instances of herpes simplex and chlamydia trachomatis as sexually transmitted diseases (*Public Health Laboratory Service Communicable Disease Report*, Table 7.1) showed totals of 14,067 and 29,104 in 1986. In 1990, the annual number of herpes simplex identifications (Table 13, Series MB2 No.17, England and Wales) had fallen back to 10,113 and identifications of chlamydia A had remained about the same at 30,078. In 1993, the number of herpes simplex infections listed in the same source was 12,135.

According to a review of the epidemiology of sexually transmitted diseases in England and Wales based on GUM clinic returns and laboratory reports, there were two contrasting patterns of change during the 1980s (Catchpole 1992). The number of new cases of sexually transmitted disease recorded in England and Wales increased by 21 per cent overall, mostly due to an increase in viral infections (genital warts and genital herpes) and 'non-specific' genital infection (NSGI) including chlamydia trachomatis; while the numbers of cases of gonorrhoea, syphilis and trichomoniasis declined. The greatest increase was presentations of genital warts (resulting from HPV infection) which rose by 130 per cent for males and 190 per cent for females; presentations of genital herpes simplex rose by 50 per cent for males and 110 per cent for females. Prior to 1988, however, primary and recurrent cases of genital warts and genital herpes simplex were not reported separately, and repeat attendances as a result of recurrent symptoms will have resulted in some cases being counted more than once in the year, thus inflating the figures. The commentator on epidemiological trends in STDs over the decade suggested that the increased proportion of viral infections diagnosed in GUM clinics might be:

> partly the result of increased ascertainment due to growing public and professional concern about genital herpes and the association of genital warts with cervical cancer, as well as increased numbers of patients with recurrent disease. The recurrence of genital herpes and genital warts in patients with HIV infection may also have contributed to increased case numbers in the latter part of the decade ... However, the increase in these conditions is unlikely to be accounted for by these factors alone.
>
> (Catchpole 1992)

Knowledge that suppressive treatment was available might have encouraged people with recurrent HSV symptoms to make repeat visits to the clinics.

There was a significant increase in the proportion of females seen in GUM clinics over the decade (though in 1990 male cases still outnumbered female cases for most conditions). This will have resulted partly from the decline in new cases of gonorrhoea and syphilis particularly associated with male homosexuals, and a greater proportional increase in new female cases (37 per cent) than for males (2 per cent) which was associated with greater increases in presentations of genital herpes, genital warts and NSGI among women. Although some of the increased female attendance may have resulted from a greater willingness on the part of women to attend GUM clinics, and thus a shift from other health service outlets, particularly general practice, there was also a greater increase in laboratory reports of genital chlamydia and genital herpes infections among females than males. Catchpole (1992) suggested that the increase in genital chlamydia and viral STDs among women was of particular concern as the serious sequelae of these conditions are predominantly seen among females – chlamydia infections being associated with pelvic inflammatory disease and ophthalmia neonatorum, and genital warts with cervical carcinoma and cervical intraepithelial neoplasia (CIN).

Clinical identification of genital herpes simplex is not normally accompanied by accurate serological typing so that the description 'genital' refers to the site of infection rather than the type of HSV infection, which could be either HSV-1 or HSV-2. There is considerable cross-reactivity between HSV-1 and HSV-2 antibodies, and wide variations between rates of seroprevalence have been found in studies of different populations using a variety of laboratory techniques. No commercial tests available reliably distinguish between HSV-1 and HSV-2 (Slomka 1996). It is only in recent years that accurate serotyping has been possible and provided increased knowledge of the prevalence of HSV-1 and HSV-2 infection and understanding of genital herpes simplex. Mertz (1993) suggests that the problems of accurate virus typing were resolved in the early 1980s with the development of monoclonal antibodies for typing virus isolates and particularly with the development of more reliable type-specific serologic assays such as the Western blot and immunodot assays.

According to Corey, who, with a colleague in Washington, developed a particular Western blot assay test which was then used to carry out a number of serosurveys on different populations, 'genital HSV infections appear to be rapidly acquired in the third decade of life', acquisition rates averaging 2.4 per cent yearly (Corey 1994). Corey quotes a study by Christenson et al. (1992) in which the seroprevalence of HSV-2 in Scandinavian women increased from 2 per cent to 25 per cent between the ages of 15 and 30 years. This author (Corey 1994) lists a range of prevalence rates for HSV-2 among various population groups in the USA and UK: 23 per cent among a Seattle family medical clinic population, 32 per cent for male and 43 per cent for female STD clinic patients in King County; 27 per cent and 37 per cent respectively for male and female heterosexual STD clinic patients. Another commentator on the epidemiology of genital herpes simplex infections (Mertz 1993) also suggests that seroprevalence rates vary widely according to the population studied and quotes rates of 22 per cent of women attending a Pennsylvania family planning clinic population (Breinig et al. 1990), 32 per cent of pregnant women consulting private obstetricians in a study based in Stanford (Kulhanjian et al. 1992), 46 per cent of women attending a STD clinic in Seattle (Koutsky et al. 1992). Prevalence rates for HSV-2 infection in STD clinic populations in Australia have been found to be around 40 per cent (Cunningham et al. 1993) and, in one study of heterosexual men, to have increased between 1985 and 1991 from 41 per cent to 65 per cent (Bassett et al. 1994).

The prevalence of HSV-2, as with HSV-1, increases with increasing age. Two recently published seroepidemiologic studies in the USA have demonstrated that HSV-2 antibody prevalence also varies with gender, race, income and educational levels and number of sexual partners. One of these studies (Johnson et al. 1989) tested more than 4,000 serum samples obtained in the late 1970s from US adults who were in the National Health and Nutrition Examination Survey (NHANES). In subjects under 15 years, less than 1 per cent had antibodies to HSV-2, but the proportion rose to 20 per cent in subjects between 30 and 44 years. In subjects who were 30 years old at least, HSV-2 antibody was found in approximately 20 per cent of white males, 25 per cent of white females, over 40 per cent of black males and over 60 per cent of black females. In a recent random household survey of unmarried adults in San Francisco (the AMEN study), HSV-2 antibody was again found more commonly in women than in men (in every age group except the oldest), and in blacks and Hispanics more commonly than non-Hispanic whites (Siegel et al. 1992). Both studies found that there was a positive association between detection of HSV-2 antibody and lower income or education level.

In 1989, Ades et al. published the results of a study of sera taken from 3,533 women on their first attendance at an antenatal clinic in a West London Hospital in 1980 and 1981 and later examined for HSV antibodies. The aim of the study was to determine the prevalence of HSV-1 and HSV-2 antibodies in this population of pregnant women and to estimate the incidence of primary infection from age specific prevalence rates. An overall prevalence rate of 78 per cent for HSV-1 and 10 per cent for HSV-2 was found, with considerable variations according to ethnic group, age, social class and marital status. The seroprevalence of HSV-1 antibody was relatively high in this study (Ades et al. 1989), giving little support to the suggestion (Corey and Spear 1986) that HSV-1 seroprevalence rates in industrialised countries are falling. HSV-1 seroprevalence rates increased with age (from an average of 75 per cent under 20 years to 91 per cent at 35 years and over), and showed some variation according to ethnicity, with black women born in the Caribbean or Africa being most likely to be seropositive (92 per cent, 96 per cent). There was also a strong association with social class – women in the non-manual group had rates between 6 per cent and 24 per cent lower than those in the manual group when rates were standardised within ethnic groups for age and marital status; for example, white UK women in the non-manual group had a rate of 75 per cent compared with a rate of 87 per cent in the manual group.

HSV-2 seroprevalence was also found to vary, in particular, according to age (increasing from an average of 4 per cent under 20 years to 19 per cent for those 35 years or older), marital status, with a rate among white single women almost twice that of married or cohabiting women (12 per cent as opposed to 6 per cent), and ethnicity (Ades et al. 1989). The study found a seroprevalence rate of 3 per cent among Asian women, 7 per cent among white women, 15 per cent among black women from the UK, 33 per cent among black Caribbean women and 37 per cent among black African women. The authors suggest that the difference between the lower HSV-2 seroprevalence rate in this study and the higher rates published in studies carried out in the USA could be associated with differences in laboratory methods. However, a recent commentary by Slomka (1996) on the seroepidemiology of genital herpes implies that such a difference is in line with an overall difference in levels of infection between the USA and UK. This author sums up the situation:

> The seroprevalence in STD clinic attenders is higher than that in samples of the general adult population in the same country or city. The seroprevalence of HSV-2 in STD clinic attenders is higher in Seattle than in London.
>
> (Slomka 1996)

THE BIOMEDICAL CONTEXT

The term 'herpes' refers to a category of viruses known as the human herpes viruses. This group includes varicella zoster which causes chicken pox and shingles (herpes zoster), the Epstein-Barr virus which is the cause of glandular fever, cytomegalovirus (CMV), the recently named human herpes virus 6 (HHV6) whose medical significance is currently unclear, as well as the *herpes simplex* virus

(HSV). As we saw in the preceding section, there are two very similar types of HSV, HSV-1 and HSV-2, and infection at some time in life with one or the other version is extremely common. The virus is a minute micro-organism (basic form of life) containing deoxyribonucleic acid (DNA) which is the genetic material. The DNA of HSV types 1 and 2 is slightly different, as are some of the glycoproteins on the outer surface of the virus which help it attach to human cells. However, there is no difference in the infection produced, and the resulting antibodies, although distinguishable, are very similar.

Infection occurs when the virus enters the body via the epithelial cells of the skin if there is a cut or break, or through the mucous membranes (such the lining of the mouth or genitals). The commonest infection sites are around the lips or mouth commonly called 'cold sores', in the genital or anal area, and on a finger (herpetic whitlow). HSV-1 is the more prevalent and the most likely cause of 'cold sores' as it has a preference for expression on the face. It is usually transmitted by kissing when the virus is active (see below), many people being infected by relatives in childhood. Prior infection with HSV-1 provides some, but not complete, immunity against HSV-2 (Mertz 1993; Corey 1994). 'Genital herpes', that is infection in the genital area, can be caused by either HSV-1 through orogenital sex, or by HSV-2, but recurrences are more likely with HSV-2 infection. The percentage of genital infections caused by HSV-1 is from 20 to 60 per cent of new cases in Britain (Patel, Cowan and Barton 1997). The variation is 'probably reflecting the variable popularity of orogenital sex in different communities' (Mindel and Carney 1991: 4). Infections on the lips or around the mouth with HSV-2 can also result from orogenital sex. HSV-2 can in fact occur in a number of non-genital areas, the most common of these being the thighs, buttocks, breasts, hands or fingers. Infection at these sites is likely to be the result of 'direct inoculation' at the time of first contracting the virus (ibid.: 29). Auto-inoculation is thought to be possible during the primary infection, but not after that time when the individual has developed antibodies (Mindel and Carney 1991: 9, 71); that is, the individual can not re-infect him or herself at another site.

The first episode of symptoms usually occurs between two and twenty days after contact with the source of infection. Initial symptoms are likely to be tingling, itching, burning and discomfort, with swollen glands and development of a red area of skin. A number of fluid-filled blisters (vesicles), 'ranging from one or two to several dozen' (Mindel and Carney 1991: 13), appear on the inflamed area. These vesicles burst, or otherwise resolve, after a few days and may leave weeping painful sores (ulcers), depending on where they occur. These ulcers may take a week to ten days to dry, scab over (if on the outer skin) and heal in the first symptom episode. In women, a vaginal discharge may also occur due to inflammation of the cervix if infection has occurred at that site, and urination can be painful if the urine touches open sores. Men may experience a discharge from the urethra and pain on urination if vesicles occur inside the urethral canal. Some people do not develop blisters, but experience a small ulcer in the form of one or more cuts or cracks in the skin. Sometimes crops of blisters develop every few days for a week or more. Flu-like symptoms can be experienced such as fever, and generalised aches and pains, and may leave the person feeling depressed and run-down. The severity and range of symptoms varies considerably, with some people experiencing minimal symptoms that they barely notice, and others feeling quite ill. The whole episode may last anything from one to three or four weeks. Infection in the perianal area or inside the anus is likely to result in pain around the anus, an anal discharge, bleeding and pain on defecation, and feelings of being generally unwell and debilitated. The sores may take rather longer to heal in this area, and infection is a possibility.

After this primary episode, indicative of infection with HSV, the virus remains in the body, travelling up the nerve route to the ganglion – usually either the sacral (lower half of the body) or the trigeminal ganglion (face), where it will live harmlessly in the nerve cells but cannot be reached by the immune system. It will be in a dormant state unless reactivated, when the virus will travel down the nerve again to produce symptoms on the skin. Such recurrences (symptomatic episodes) are nearly always shorter and less severe than the primary episode, on average lasting a few days to a week. The natural history of the condition in a particular person is extremely variable. Some people will never have a recurrence, others only one or two a year, whereas others may have them frequently; in many, the frequency and severity of recurrences reduces over the years, whereas in some others they remain about the same. Often, the experience of recurrences is periodic and there may be long periods without any sign of the infection, followed by a time of increased activity. The first signs of a recurrence are often warning or prodromal symptoms such as a burning, tingling or itching sensation in the skin, or neuralgia (pain along a nerve) like a stabbing pain which may be in the groin, buttock, genital area, thigh or back of the leg in the case of infection in the lower half of the body. An individual at the start of a recurrence may also feel 'off-colour'. These warning signs tend to occur a few hours or more before any signs appear on the skin, and for some people are more uncomfortable than the blisters themselves, which are likely to be in a small group. Not everyone has prodromal symptoms and not every warning sign is followed by a full-blown recurrence: the redness and blisters may come and go in a short time or not occur at all.

The site of recurrent symptoms is usually the same as in the primary episode, although symptoms tend to recur on the external genitalia or the perianal skin rather than internally. Sometimes, the symptoms occur on the thighs or buttocks even if this was not the site of the primary episode. When the virus reactivates in the nerve cells of the sacral ganglia it may proceed down an adjacent branch of the nerve to one leading to the genitals. There are a number of physical and psychological factors, any of which may act as triggers for reactivation, and in a predisposing combination of circumstances, lead to a recurrence of HSV symptoms. A large number of research studies (discussed in Chapter 5) have attempted to unravel the mystery of the combination of associated factors and determine predictors of recurrences. Exposure to strong sunlight is one such trigger, and individuals who get herpes simplex symptoms on an exposed part of their body may be helped by protecting that part with sun block. Illness, fatigue from lack of sleep or intense activity, being run-down, and in women, menstruation, may also trigger a recurrence of symptoms. It appears that friction and damage to the skin around the genitals during sexual intercourse may be another precipitating factor. In some people, stress and anxiety are associated with recurrences, although it can be difficult to know which comes first and triggers the other, the recurrence or the associated stress. It is also suggested that there are dietary deficiencies which may predispose to recurrent symptoms. Clearly, anything which lowers the immune system's ability to keep the activity of the virus in check could be associated with recurrent symptoms.

While is not difficult to recognise the classic symptoms and signs of an obvious episode of herpes simplex, it is important to stress how very variable the signs, symptoms and natural history of this common self-limiting condition can be. In some cases, symptoms of the condition may be so minor – passing discomfort, a small area of redness, a tiny blister or two, or a small break in the skin, that they go unrecognised. Termed 'inapparent' (Mindel and Carney 1991: 18) and 'subclinical' (Corey 1994), evidence has accumulated in recent years that the majority of people who are seropositive for HSV have unrecognised infection. A study involving nearly 800 women randomly selected from a STD clinic population in USA (Hook, Cannon, Nahmias et al. 1992) found 43 per cent had acquired HSV-2 infection but two-thirds had no history of genital ulcers and no evidence on examination in the clinic. Two studies (Langenberg, Benedetti, Jenkins et al. 1989; Frenkel, Garratty, Shen et al. 1993) investigating apparently asymptomatic HSV-2 found that patients could be taught to recognise signs and symptoms of a recurrence. Corey (1994) suggests that of the proportion of the population who are seropositive for HSV-2, 80 per cent actually have symptomatic not asymptomatic genital herpes, (with 20 per cent recognised symptomatic and 60 per cent unrecognised symptomatic) and only 20 per cent are truly subclinical. Mertz (1993) suggests that from 10 per cent to 40 per cent of individuals with genital HSV infections are aware of the condition and that atypical lesions are a factor in undiagnosed genital herpes simplex. In another study of STD clinic patients (Koutsky, Stevens, Holmes et al. 1992), typical external lesions were seen in only two-thirds of women with positive HSV cultures; in the other third, HSV was isolated from atypical lesions, or from the cervix, vulva or rectum without signs or symptoms being present. Corey (1994) has commented that:

> Genital herpes probably is one of the most difficult STD to diagnose. The clinical spectrum is diverse, and because of this, clinical diagnosis has reasonable specificity but poor sensitivity. The manifestations of genital herpes vary widely among individuals and even between episodes within an individual, making laboratory confirmation often a necessity.

If the first episode of symptoms goes unrecognised, and the virus is thereafter largely dormant, the individual may be completely unaware that they are infected. It is nonetheless possible to have a recurrence at some stage which is more noticeable and results in a diagnosis. This may happen years after the initial infection and may result in the individual becoming suspicious of his or her sexual partner's faithfulness, or vice versa, leading to accusations and mutual distress.

In the Western world, herpes simplex is the commonest cause of ulcers in the genital area. However, there are other causes and for this reason, among others, it can be important to obtain a definitive diagnosis. Other infections which may cause sores are syphilis, which usually causes a single painless ulcer, sexually transmitted diseases occurring in the tropics, such as chancroid which causes painful genital ulcers which do not resolve without antibiotics; candida and trichomoniasis may sometimes cause superficial sores, and the skin burrows of the scabies parasite might appear like herpes sores. Trauma, some skin diseases and rare syndromes might also be confused with herpes simplex. Confirmation that HSV is the cause of genital signs and symptoms is made by taking a swab or scraping from an ulcer or blister which is then sent for laboratory analysis. The specimen is then either tissue-cultured (a technique which requires a number of days for cells to grow in the culture medium), or submitted to antigen analysis, which enables specific components of the virus to be identified and produces a result within a few hours. This latter technique has become more accurate in recent years and it is now possible with some tests to determine whether the infection is HSV-1 or HSV-2. However, swab tests depend on the presence of active HSV. In recurrent episodes, viral isolation is only 50 per cent sensitive (Corey 1994): although obvious lesions may be present, the individual's immune response may eradicate the infectious virus within a few days. It is possible to confirm the presence of HSV nucleic acid in such lesions using a polymase chain reaction assay, but this test is expensive and not normally available. In an individual with suspected HSV infection, but without any current signs, a blood test can be performed to check for antibodies. However, unless the test is able to distinguish between HSV-1 and HSV-2, as in the type-specific serologic essays developed in the USA (see earlier section), the information that there has been contact at some stage with HSV is not very useful when such infection is so widespread.

Infection occurs when there is direct skin to skin contact with the site of viral shedding, which happens when the virus is active at the skin's surface, rather than dormant in the nerve cells.

As a general rule, a person is only likely to be infective as long as any symptoms or signs are present. This means that infectivity is a risk from the start of the prodrome (warning symptoms) to the healing of the last ulcer.

(Wellcome Australia: *Genital Herpes: A Facts Book* p. 5)

When there are herpetic symptoms around the mouth (cold sores), it is necessary to avoid kissing or oral sex in order to prevent passing on the infection to someone who is not infected already. In particular, it is important when cold sores are present not to kiss small babies (whose immune systems are not fully developed until around six months). When sores or blisters occur elsewhere, it is necessary to prevent another individual's direct contact with them to avoid the risk of passing on the infection. If these signs are in the anogenital area, avoidance of sexual contact is necessary. Sometimes protection can be achieved by use of a condom if it covers the area that is shedding virus or is exposed to the virus. In a very small number of women, sores occur only on the cervix, where they cannot be seen. Mostly, these women would experience typical symptoms, but some may be unaware that they are infected. In at least one study (Mertz, Benedetti and Ashley 1992), the risk of male-to-female transmission was found to be greater than female-to-male transmission.

It is possible for the virus to be present on the skin's surface without any obvious signs or symptoms. The risk of asymptomatic shedding appears to be influenced by the virus type, the risk being higher in the genital area with HSV-2, and the temporal proximity to the primary episode, the risk being highest in the subsequent three to twelve months (Koelle et al. 1992). In a recent prospective cohort study by Wald et al. (1995), the median number of days during which asymptomatic viral shedding was recorded was 1.1 per cent, with none at all detected in about half the women in the study. Women with frequent recurrences (more than twelve a year), were more likely to have asymptomatic viral shedding. It is known that asymptomatic shedding of HSV occurs in men and that it appears to be responsible for more than half the cases of sexually trans-mitted genital HSV infections, but the site and frequency of asymptomatic shedding has been difficult to determine (Mertz 1993). In a series of studies in pregnant and non-pregnant women, the risk of asymptomatic shedding from the cervix or vulva has ranged from about 0.4 per cent to 1.3 per cent per day (ibid.). In a study of 144 couples, only one of whom was infected with HSV-2, the annual risk of transmission was found to be 17 per cent in couples in whom the female was susceptible and 4 per cent in couples where the male partner was susceptible. The risk in women was over three times as high in those who did not have HSV-1 antibodies as compared with those who did (ibid.).

Most genital infections are passed on inadvertently, and transmission of HSV during sexual activity in periods of unrecognised lesions or subclinical reactivation of the virus is an important factor in the spread of infection. The indications are that it is the latently infected carrier with an unrecognised condition who accounts for the widespread prevalence of this infection (Corey 1993). In people with recognised recurrences, a small risk of transmission will remain both during periods of asymptomatic shedding and during the period shortly before lesions are recognised (Mertz 1993). Barrier methods of contraception are an important approach to the prevention of transmission until a safe and effective HSV vaccine is in general use (Corey 1994).

While herpes simplex is essentially a minor, self-limiting condition, it can cause occasional and rare complications, particularly in association with the primary episode. The most frequently encountered complication is difficulty with urination during a primary episode in women. If blisters or open sores are inside the urethra, or on the inner side of the labia minora or around the urethra in a woman, urination may cause intense pain, and this may result in urinary retention. The condition may be eased by attempting to dilute the urine, urinating in a bath of warm water, or separating the labia to stop the urine coming in contact with the sores. Pain relief may be sufficient to encourage urination to occur in the normal way. A condition known as sacral radiculomyelopathy, a neurological complication in which the HSV infection may affect the nerve cells at the base of the spine, also causes urinary problems. This condition only occurs in primary episodes and is more usually associated with severe perianal infection. Apart from problems with urination and defaecation, it is associated with pain in the back of the thigh or buttocks, decreased skin sensitivity around the anal or genital area, and, in men, problems with obtaining an erection. The condition lasts two to three weeks, recovers spontaneously and does not result in long-term neurological problems. If it results in complete inability to pass urine, a catheter may have to be passed into the bladder (either through the urethra or through the suprapubic area) to drain the urine.

The herpes simplex virus (HSV) may on rare occasions cause

infections other than the very common 'cold sores' or typical genital ulcers. Infection in the eye mostly involves the conjunctiva, and is likely to be very painful. Without treatment, the cornea could be damaged from ulceration with resultant loss of vision; however, early treatment with an antiviral agent is very successful. Herpes simplex is among the many bacteria and viruses which can cause meningitis. Such infection, if it occurs, is most likely to be associated with a severe primary genital episode; however, the meningitis is comparatively mild and short lived, recovering completely within a few days without long term neurological consequences. It would be treated with an antiviral agent such as acyclovir. Encephalis is not so easily diagnosed or treated, but the infection is extremely rare. In people with severely compromised immune systems, HSV infection can occur in the oesophagus and internal organs. This is a serious problem which occurs in people with HIV/AIDS, who often require long-term antiviral therapy.

The UK Herpes Association's *Herpes Simplex: A Guide* rightly suggests that 'pregnancy and childbirth is the most sensitive and worrying issue connected with Herpes simplex'. Carmack and Prober (1993) acknowledge that because the prognosis is still not good for the very small number of neonates who do acquire HSV infection:

> Such apprehension is justified for a disease that is difficult to predict, problematic to diagnose, and associated with high morbidity and mortality despite the availability of antiviral therapy.

Anxiety and concern have certainly been heightened by the way the subject has been treated in the media, as discussed earlier. Any significant risk is confined to a situation in which a woman is infected and has a primary episode after conception. If this happens in the first twenty weeks of pregnancy there is an increased risk of spontaneous abortion, stillbirth and congenital malformations (Whitley 1993a), as with other viral infections. If this happens shortly before birth, so that the woman is suffering a primary episode and the virus is active and being shed from the cervix and birth canal, this carries a 33–50 per cent chance of the baby being infected (Whitley 1993a; Mertz 1993) with significant morbidity and mortality. This situation is very unusual; however, it could happen if the woman's partner was infected with HSV-2 and she was not, and the infection was passed on at this time. In this situation, assuming it was recognised, a Caesarean section delivery would be recommended to bypass the birth canal.

In a woman with a history of recurrent HSV symptoms on the genitalia prior to conception, the risk to the baby from the infection is very low, virtually nil, assuming that the baby is 'in full receipt of its mother's antibodies', according to the UK Herpes Association (1993a), 'remote' according to Mindel and Carney (1991: 54). Whether the maternal infection is primary or recurrent is the most important factor influencing the acquisition of infection by the baby. In a primary infection, large amounts of virus are excreted for as long as two weeks; in a recurrent infection, virus shedding lasts for about three days. Furthermore, with recurrent infection, the mother's antibodies will play a protective role which will last for a number of months after birth, both reducing the likelihood of infection and the severity of the infection if it occurs. Two additional factors influencing the possibility of neonatal infection are the duration of ruptured membranes – the longer the membranes are ruptured the greater the probability of ascending infection – and the use of a foetal scalp monitor (Whitley 1993a). In fact, the majority of women giving birth do so carrying antibodies to HSV due to past infection with types 1 or 2 or both. Whitley (1993a) argued that 'protective mechanisms for the foetus must be operative', since many babies are born safely to women who will have acquired genital HSV infection before their pregnancy, and the occurrence of neonatal HSV infection is far less common than would be projected from the prevalence of genital HSV infection among adults of child-bearing age in general. The routine use of Caesarean section simply because a woman has a history of genital HSV symptoms is clearly unjustified and no longer generally recommended, because the risk to the baby is very low, and Caesarean section carries some risk for the mother.

There is some degree of controversy, however, about the most appropriate management of a situation where there is a recurrence of genital HSV symptoms at the time of delivery. A very small but serious risk to the baby has to be weighed up against the risk to the mother of a Caesarean section. Additional factors which enter the equation are that a Caesarean section delivery does not always eliminate the risk of infection (Stone et al. 1989), and the position of lesions which are not in the birth canal but on the labia, for instance, so that the baby is less likely to come into direct contact with them. In the early 1980s in the USA, management of women with a history of genital HSV symptoms included weekly cervical cultures, followed by an automatic Caesarean section delivery if the culture was positive. This protocol has since been abandoned by the American College of Obstetricians and Gynecologists and new guidelines substituted (ACOG 1988), because the previous strategy was 'fruitless' (Carmack and Prober 1993). It takes several days to get the results (isolate the virus in tissue culture) by which time the mother may no longer be excreting virus, and because more than 70 per cent of women giving birth to infants with neonatal HSV report no signs or symptoms of HSV infection, nor a sexual partner with evidence of genital HSV infection. Thus, such screening missed most of the women at risk of passing on the infection. However:

> The cost of screening all women at delivery currently appears unjustified, and there is no practical, inexpensive method currently available to identify the women at highest risk of transmission, those at risk of first-episode genital herpes at term.
>
> (Mertz 1993)

A large-scale prospective investigation reported in 1991 (Brown et al. 1991) assessed the risk factors associated with neonatal HSV acquisition. The study involved culturing the cervix and external genitalia of 15,923 pregnant women in early labour who had no evidence on admission to the labour unit. In those women in whom HSV was isolated from the genital tract cultures (56, 0.35 per cent), fifty-two subsequently had serologic tests to find out if the infection was a primary infection or a reactivation. Neonatal HSV developed in six of eighteen babies (33 per cent) born to seronegative mothers, but only one of thirty-four infants (3 per cent) born to seropositive mothers: that is, ten times fewer. The reported rates of neonatal HSV infections in the USA appear to vary considerably: 0.04 per cent in the Brown et al. (1991) study, 0.003 per cent according to the study by Roberts et al. (1995) (3 per 100,000 births), and 0.029–0.02 per cent (1 per 3,500–5,000 deliveries) according to Whitley (1993a). In the UK (excluding Wales), the reported rate of neonatal infection over the ten-year period 1976–85 was fourteen cases per year (2–3 per 100,000 births) (Ades et al. 1989). Antiviral agents (vidarabine and azyclovir) have improved the prognosis for infants with HSV infection: according to Whitley (1993a) infants with localised infection survive; in those with encephalitis, the mortality is 15 per cent, with 50 per cent developing normally thereafter; 50 per cent of infants with disseminated infection survive and of these about 85 per cent develop normally thereafter. Where the infection is recognised and therapy instituted early, fewer infants progress from localised skin involvement to more serious infections.

A neonate is also at risk from HSV infection after birth, particularly if it has no protection from maternal HSV antibodies – that is, if its mother was *not* previously infected with either type of HSV. Whitley suggests that hospital staff with current herpetic whitlows should not care for newborns, and individuals with recurrences on the face or elsewhere on the body should take appropriate precautions including careful hand washing. A significant proportion of neonatal infections are caused by HSV-1: nearly 30 per cent according to Whitley (1993a), 50 per cent according to the British Paediatric Surveillance Unit's statistics.

Medical treatment of HSV infection was advanced greatly in the early 1980s by the discovery that acyclovir ('Zovirax' produced by Wellcome) stopped the replication of the virus and was 'specific, safe and highly efficacious' (Mindel and Carney 1991: 47). It is possible to reduce significantly the severity of the primary episode, and if subsequently there are frequent recurrences, largely to suppress the activity of the virus. It is not possible to cure the infection because the virus cannot be eliminated from the body, but specific antiviral therapy has revolutionised possible medical intervention for this condition. Treating a primary episode of HSV infection with acyclovir tablets (200 mg five times daily) is standard practice nowadays (Whitley and Gnann 1992), and very effective if it is started within two or three days after blisters first develop. The treatment reduces symptoms including pain, fever, headaches, and flu-like symptoms, shortening the duration of symptoms and the time during which there is viral shedding and until the blisters heal (Whitley and Gnann 1992). If the treatment is started after the blisters have started to heal, it is less effective. Occasionally, hospital admission is recommended for a person suffering a very severe first episode with urinary retention or meningitis and acyclovir is given by injection.

Acyclovir tablets have also been prescribed to treat each recurrence but its efficacy is minimal, reducing the time for healing by a marginal amount – no more than one day if the treatment is started early in the episode (Whitley and Gnann 1992). The drug is also available as a cream to apply to lesions, but again the evidence is that it makes very little difference and there are other topical applications such as an ointment containing the anaesthetic xylocaine which are considerably cheaper and possibly more helpful. Many people with recurrent symptoms of HSV infection do not require medical intervention and find various ways (including ice packs and saline bathing – see Chapter 3) to relieve the relatively minor and short-lived discomfort. However, suppressive or prophylactic treatment which involves taking tablets every day, is available and was shown in a succession of clinical trials in the 1980s (Mindel 1993) to be effective in preventing recurrences in the genital area. Selection of patients for long-term suppressive therapy is based primarily on the frequency of recurrences, with those who have more than eight episodes a year definitely being considered and those with less than six not normally being candidates. Mindel (1993) suggests that patients who have between six and eight recurrences a year 'may be suitable for suppression if the recurrences are severe, prolonged, or causing profound psychological or psychosexual problems', and that time should be allowed to elapse so that the pattern of recurrences can become evident before such treatment is started. The number of tablets taken is started at a higher dose (such as 200 mg four times daily) and then reduced to the lowest number which allows the person to remain recurrence-free.

The majority of people taking suppressive acyclovir either have no recurrences or very few minor, brief episodes. The treatment also reduces prodromal symptoms, scars or marks left on the skin from previous recurrences and psychosexual disturbance. However, studies have shown that asymptomatic viral shedding may still occur (at rates of less than 1 per cent), and thus a low risk of transmission may remain (Straus et al. 1989; Bowman et al. 1990, Wald et al. 1996). A number of clinical trials have shown that if the treatment is stopped after only a few months, the recurrences return with the same frequency and severity as before; but if treatment is continued for a longer period (at least a year), the frequency of recurrences after stopping therapy can be markedly reduced. Two studies (Mindel et al. 1988; Straus et al. 1989) have shown that there is statistically significant difference between the number of recurrences before and after one to two years of suppressive therapy, though whether the reduction is due to the natural history of the condition or the treatment is not clear. Treatment should be interrupted on a yearly basis to reassess the need for continuing suppression.

Acyclovir is now the 'most widely prescribed and clinically

effective antiviral drug available' (Whitley and Gnann 1992). There appear to be no serious adverse side effects from long-term acyclovir therapy, and only a small risk of transient side effects such as nausea and minor skin rashes when treatment is first started.

Therapy over 5 years has been well tolerated and not associated with serious side effects or cumulative toxicity.

(Goldberg et al. 1993)

According to a report on the safety of acyclovir use 'in over 20 million persons treated worldwide over the past decade, complemented by . . . structured epidemiologic studies closely monitoring the experience of over 50,000 patients' there is a 'persuasive body of information concerning the general safety of this important therapeutic intervention' (Tilson, Engle and Andrews 1993). Acyclovir is expensive, however, and there has been a reluctance among some doctors in the UK at least to prescribe it for suppressive therapy.

It is not clear yet whether it is safe to take the drug during pregnancy (trials of oral acyclovir during late pregnancy are taking place), but it is not currently recommended. However, where acyclovir has been taken inadvertently in the early months of pregnancy, no untoward effects appear to have occurred (Spangler, Kirk and Knudson 1994).

Prior to the discovery of the action of acyclovir, a drug called idoxuridine ('Herpid'), which had marked antiviral activity against several viruses including herpes simplex, had been used but had serious systemic side effects because it affected cells other than those infected with HSV. Whereas, acyclovir is incorporated into the viral DNA in infected cells, but not the human DNA in uninfected cells. Vidarabine was the first drug licensed for systemic use as an antiviral agent and improved the outlook for treatment of herpes simplex encephalitis in immunocompromised patients and in neonatal infections. However, there were some significant clinical problems associated with its use (Whitley 1993b). Valaciclovir ('Valtrex') is a recent development from acyclovir (an L-valyl ester of acyclovir) which is well absorbed and rapidly converted to acyclovir resulting in three to fourfold higher acyclovir levels than can be achieved with oral acyclovir. (Acyclovir has low bioavailability with less than 20 per cent of the available drug being absorbed and absorption levels varying.) The implication is that the number of valaciclovir tablets taken per day for patients on suppressive therapy could be reduced. It also means that substantially higher plasma levels of acyclovir can be achieved through oral administration. Another recently developed drug for the treatment of herpes simplex and herpes zoster, which is also more efficient in terms of its bioavailability than acyclovir, is famciclovir ('Famvir', produced by SmithKline and Beecham).

The future holds the promise of a vaccine to prevent the acquisition of HSV infection in the first place (see Chapter 7). In this chapter, the sociocultural, epidemiological and medical context of the current problem of HSV infection have been reviewed. We have seen how common HSV infection is, and how, for most people who acquire it, it is not a problem at all. When it is a problem, medical intervention to relieve the symptoms is possible. We have also seen, however, the highly negative constructions put on the condition so that it has been presented in the worst possible light, and in exaggerated and scaremongering terms in the media. The burden of this image falls on the unfortunate few who suffer from their infection and have to live with it knowingly, managing intermittent symptoms and the psychosocial impact of the stigma. The following chapters will review what is known of their experiences and the psychosocial factors involved.

Chapter 2

The impact of diagnosis

This chapter will look at the impact, in physical and emotional terms, of a primary occurrence of HSV infection, its diagnosis and the implications of the condition. It will review the changing medical response to a diagnosis of HSV infection in the genital area and discuss issues involved in dealing with the impact and carrying on with life. Inevitably, the recorded representations of this impact tend to be from expressive people for whom it was very significant rather than from those for whom it was fairly inconsequential, so that it is important to bear in mind that both the physical symptoms of a first episode of HSV infection and the personal responses involved can vary greatly.

One might well wonder what kind of condition could induce its sufferers to express such a wide range of very negative feelings including shock, devastation, fear, anger, bitterness, hate, disgust, isolation, exposure, vulnerability, grief, shame, guilt, feeling unclean, tainted, or like a leper, worthless, handicapped for life, hopeless, and suicidal? Without adequate support and accurate information, a diagnosis of HSV infection can plunge the recipient into despair associated with the thought that they are stuck with the condition for life, that an intimate relationship is no longer possible, and that life is no longer worth living.

When the doctor diagnosed genital herpes I felt the carpet had been pulled from beneath me and my life was over. I desperately hoped it was all a terrible mistake.

(*Sphere*, 9(2): 16)

Together with my emotional loss the fact of having herpes and its implications struck a chord that I never knew I would feel.

Devastation would describe it adequately . . . who would want me and my herpes together?

(*Sphere*, 2(4): 12)

The following is a description of the impact of diagnosis on one man writing about his personal experience of herpes simplex in *Sphere*, the newsletter of the UK Herpes Association (HA). He had attended a STD clinic in a London hospital and the doctor had simply told him to bathe in salty water and that it was an incurable condition.

I didn't hear any more, '*incurable*', he said. I was stunned by that word, and wandered out into the busy back-street with the word ringing in my head, feeling quite numb and disconnected. Suddenly my whole perspective had changed in those few short minutes. When I did eventually find my parked car, I was in a daze, and sat for a while gripping the wheel and watching 'normal', chattering people pass by without a care in the world, hoping they didn't know what I had 'got'.

(*Sphere*, 2(4): 11)

Among accounts of their personal experiences of living with symptoms of HSV printed in *Sphere*, a proportion mentioned having suicidal feelings at some stage before coming to terms with having the condition.

I . . . was naturally devastated when first diagnosed and mentally went through some very difficult weeks and even had thoughts of suicide . . . put in touch with support groups . . . I find meeting others on a social basis a tremendous support . . . I still need M's support (from HA). If I hadn't found this two years ago, I hate to think how things would have turned out.

(*Sphere*, 9(2): 12)

Ten months ago I had my first attack of herpes. The physical symptoms were mild but psychologically I was devastated. I couldn't cope with it at all. It was the beginning of four to five months of spending a substantial part of the day in tears. No cure. I felt literally trapped, against the wall, no choice but to live this for the rest of my life. I'm a rebel – I can't stand to have no choice at all . . . so I invented one . . . I *could* commit suicide, then I wouldn't have to live with it for life! I bought the required bottle of medication I knew was lethal, put it on top of my cupboard and felt much freer. I'd never take it but *now* I had a choice; I had some control over my own destiny

(*Sphere*, 2(2))

The following quotations from HA membership survey questionnaires (Posner 1990) are testaments to the crucial support received on the Helpline by people recently diagnosed:

I had just been told I had HSV and was crying on the phone, but Chris was very patient . . . he was reassuring that my mental anguish was normal and he had felt the same.

Phoned just after diagnosis. Felt suicidal. Talked to someone who had 'been there' too and had come through it. Felt enormously relieved, and not alone, an outcast or a leper, etc. afterwards.

I mainly spoke to M whom I found to be so calm and reassuring that I don't know how I would have got through those early days without his endless patience.

A commentator in the HA newsletter wrote about initial contact with Association on the Helpline:

What helped more than I can say was the commonsense, down-to-earth, friendly support, and humour, I found when, sobbing, I first rang the helpline, and then later in HA 'get-togethers'.

(*Sphere*, 4(3): 12)

PRIMARY EPISODES

Descriptions of first episodes of HSV symptoms in the column of the HA's newsletter written by HA members about their personal experiences describe how painful, physically and emotionally, the condition can be.

The next few days were hell, have you ever tried to scream with your mouth shut? This is what I found myself doing with every visit to the loo. I once suffered a scorpion sting to the foot and this felt like much the same kind of agonising pain . . . I felt I was dying: my head felt muzzy and detached from the rest of my body; I found it was difficult to focus; colours seemed to swim together; I felt ill! I was shattered, totally exhausted and eventually allowed myself to be dragged to the local hospital.

(*Sphere*, 8(4): 12)

I personally feel that the emotional pain upon diagnosis, and indeed afterwards, which is experienced by many people needs to be recognised as being *very* real. I speak from personal experience here. I think people need to know that it's O.K. to have these feelings . . . They are perfectly natural and just part of the process of readjustment and getting back to living your life as you did before.

(*Sphere*, 9(3): 12)

I was very ill with my first attack: my whole body ached, I would scratch myself until I bled, and I couldn't go to the toilet without having to run some water into the bath . . . After two days I had developed lots of little spots, I looked at it in the mirror and my whole genital area was covered. By this time I was in agony, I couldn't go to the toilet without crying. I couldn't walk and I couldn't sit.

(*Sphere*, 5(1): 12)

My first attack was relatively severe. I was ill for five or six weeks but returned to work after two.

(*Sphere*, 6(3): 8)

The HA's own survey of its membership carried out in 1986 (*Sphere*, 3(2): 17) found that only one quarter of members responding reported having a primary episode lasting three weeks. In over half the replies, it was over in two weeks. The severity of the primary episode is not related to whether recurrences will occur or to the frequency of recurrences. There are estimates of the proportion of people with primary infection who will have recurrences, but these are based on people who sought medical help for the first occurrence, and since those without any recurrences or with only mild recurrences are unlikely to seek further medical intervention, the proportion is impossible to estimate at all accurately. It is known that in general, recurrences tend to become less frequent and less severe over time; and that recurrences are less likely when the primary infection on the genitals was caused by HSV-1, or on the face, by HSV-2.

IMPLICATIONS OF THE DIAGNOSIS

Diagnosis of herpes simplex infection in the genital area often brings in its wake a whole range of personal, social and sexual issues which can take the experience of the infection out of the realm of a simple, passing, medically minor and common, spontaneously regressing condition, into a major psychosocial problem in terms of adjustment to 'having' the condition. The sorts of personal and psychosexual issues which are raised by a diagnosis of herpes simplex infection are: 'How did I get it?', 'Who gave it to me?', 'Why didn't s/he protect me or tell me and allow me to protect myself?', 'What will this mean for my sexual and reproductive life?', 'Will anyone now accept me as a sexual partner?', 'How do I feel about myself now I have acquired a sexually transmitted and incurable condition?', 'What will other people think about me now that I have acquired such a condition?'.

A mediating factor between the physical expression of the condition and the individual person's experience is the meaning attached to it. On a desert island, the development of multiple sclerosis (MS) or insulin-dependent diabetes could mean disaster and the physical manifestations of the conditions would heavily influence that meaning whether or not the person knew the diagnosis and irrespective of the person's awareness of other people's attitudes to the problem. On a desert island, herpes simplex would be very much less of a problem, if a problem at all. Even with a severe first episode, the person would recover without medical help, and the meaning would be limited to immediate symptoms and the kind of interruption of normal activity which may accompany a cold or, at worst, flu. Herpes simplex is indeed a 'social' disease in that a large part of the significance and accompanying suffering is derived from its socially constructed meaning. When the condition is experienced without knowledge of the diagnosis, as it often is in its mild form, and without reference to other people, there is an absence of significance beyond the immediate sensation or inconvenience of the symptoms. The medical label, with its heavily stigmatised social meaning, changes that situation. Scambler (1984: 226) pointed to the paradox that:

> while doctors have it in their power to foist unwanted, stigmatizing identities upon their patients ... most, it seems, lack the training, motivation or time to offer sympathetic understanding and support to those they have, in worthy innocence, 'marked'.

The label 'herpes' carries a meaning wherever the symptoms are, and the occurrence of symptoms in the genital region carries an additional layer of meaning (as we have seen in the previous chapter). This meaning can be the cause of very considerable anxiety and emotional distress when the condition is diagnosed. Carney et al. (1994) reported recently on the results of a study which appeared to demonstrate that:

> The diagnosis of a first episode of genital herpes has a profound emotional effect on patients. If they do not have recurrent episodes, their emotional state improves.

The study used the General Health Questionnaire (GHQ), the Hospital Anxiety and Depression Scale (HADQ), Illness Attitude Scales and Illness Concern, and found at the first visit, that the primary herpes group of patients were significantly more concerned about their illness than either the GUM or Dermatology control groups, and that a higher proportion of the primary herpes group (62 per cent) were classifiable as GHQ 'cases' than in either of the other two groups (52 per cent of Dermatology controls and 34 per cent of GUM controls). No significant differences between the three groups were found in relation to depression scores or with respect to the 'quality or frequency of their sexual intercourse'. The proportion of primary herpes patients who were classifiable as GHQ or HADQ 'cases' reduced significantly, as did the illness concern scores, by three months later. Among those without recurrences, 73 per cent initially classified as GHQ cases became non-cases three months later; likewise 55 per cent of those classified as anxiety 'cases' became non-cases, and their illness concern scores were significantly lower. However, those who did have recurrences remained as concerned as they had been initially and there were no significant changes in the proportion defined as cases.

These results led Carney and colleagues (1994) to question the suggestion that it is the emotional state of the patient with newly diagnosed HSV infection which leads to recurrences (Goldmeier et al. 1988; see also the discussion 'Research studies of the relationship between psychosocial factors and recurrences' in Chapter 5). They argued that it is the physical recurrences which lead to the emotional state and that it is not possible to predict who will have recurrences from their psychological profile at the first visit.

> Recurrences may be independent of mood per se, but in themselves can have a damaging effect on the individual's well-being.
>
> (Carney et al. 1994)

They concluded that:

Clinicians need to acknowledge that not only may patients with a first episode of genital herpes be experiencing an acute and debilitating physical illness, but also that its diagnosis may precipitate further emotional reactions.

(Carney et al. 1994)

In view of the high incidence of psychological morbidity (as assessed on the GHQ) among the primary herpes simplex patients in the above study at their first clinic attendance, the finding of a Dutch study (Stronks et al. 1993), that patients with genital herpes symptoms judged themselves retrospectively as having developed more psychological complaints compared to the premorbid situation than did patients with gonorrhoea, and tended to judge themselves as having fewer psychological complaints prior to the infection, is interesting. The study authors suggested that this finding might be the result of 'response-shift bias' in which the perceptions of previous levels of functioning by patients with HSV changed due to their current confrontation with the 'incurability' of their infection.

Sometimes, the emotional reaction to a diagnosis of herpetic infection in the genital area is delayed. If the person involved has caught the infection from their partner, the possible implications of the diagnosis may only be faced at a point where the relationship is failing or ends, and the individual is faced with the prospect of finding another partner. There is some evidence that it is the perceived consequences of the condition in terms of negotiating sexual relationships which is the cause of the most upset. As part of a study by Keller, Jadack and Mims (1991) investigating the experience of recurrent genital symptoms of HSV infection, the sixty participants were asked about disease-related stressors. Respondents identified a range of from one to seventeen 'stressors' with a mean of 7.1 stressors per respondent. Most (73.9 per cent) stressors mentioned related to the consequences of the condition; others related to the symptoms and identification of recurrences (6.3 per cent), the lack of cure and unpredictability of recurrences (9.9 per cent), anger and guilt about contracting the infection (4.5 per cent) and misinformation and lack of support (3.1 per cent). Among the consequence stressors, fear of telling a new sexual partner (mentioned by 58.3 per cent), and possible transmission to a sexual partner, were the most frequently mentioned, as well as fear of intimate relationships, loss of sexual spontaneity, concerns about its effect upon health, transmission to a baby, and about others' reactions. Nearly all (96.7 per cent) participants in this study experienced a stressor relating to assumed consequences of having the condition. Less than a third of the sample (30 per cent) identified symptoms of the condition as a stressor. All the stressors which were reported as the 'most-upsetting' or 'second-most-upsetting' (by at least 3 per cent of participants) were related to the consequences of the disease.

THE MEDICAL RESPONSE

In the past, many doctors have undoubtedly been somewhat dismissive of the suffering associated with herpes simplex – whether physical or psychological – probably because of the self-limiting and usually minor nature of the condition in biomedical terms. The following is an account of an example of such treatment in a hospital clinic, reported in *Sphere* (5(1): 12):

> A doctor came in. Her exact words were 'Oh, as we thought, you've got herpes'. I had never heard of it before in my life. I asked what it was and how to clear it up. She said 'It's a virus and it's incurable. I'll give you something to dilute your urine so it won't be so painful'. That was all the help and information I received. I came out of the hospital crying my eyes out and thinking I only had six months to live!

It would be generally accepted practice now in a GUM or Sexual Health clinic to treat a primary episode of HSV infection producing severe symptoms in the genital area with acyclovir tablets in order to reduce the severity of the symptoms and their duration.

In recent years there has been a greater awareness of the need to pay attention to the information and support needs for newly diagnosed patients and those troubled by recurrences. In a letter to the editor of *Genitourinary Medicine*, Kinghorn (1992) argued that 'to provide effective management of genital herpes, physicians must address both the medical and psychosocial needs of their patients'. When they were first diagnosed patients 'should be educated about the nature, features and transmission of their infection and individually assessed to determine its likely psychosocial impact'. Patients troubled by frequent or severe recurrences might need 'additional counselling and support'. Educational sessions could help prevent the spread of the condition, Kinghorn argued. Furthermore:

Effective reassurance and counselling, together with optimal medical management of symptoms, can help reduce the frequency of recurrences and allow patients relief from the psychological distress of genital herpes.

Mindel (1993) writes of 'clinical and psychological management of genital herpes' and addresses 'psychological and psychosexual morbidity' as a part of the management plan, suggesting that:

Counselling and psychological support following first episode genital herpes should continue as long as required. Discussing some of the more emotive issues may need to be postponed until the patient has recovered from the acute episode.

While specialists may have altered their approach to the management of HSV infection in the genital area over the last decade or so, the situation among practitioners in general may be less changed. A letter from a venereologist, formerly GP, to the *New Zealand Medical Journal* (Dayan 1994) explaining the role of the New Zealand Herpes Foundation and the need for the Herpes Helpline suggests that:

The psychological effects of genital herpes have been underestimated by the medical profession in the past and often we as doctors, have had little or no training in sexual history taking or sexual counselling as undergraduates. The feedback from people seeking further information or help indicates that many doctors have little appreciation of the psychological impact a diagnosis of HSV has on a person's life.

This author records that the experiences of counsellors on the Helpline indicates how 'many patients diagnosed with HSV are not receiving optimum management from their doctor', and argues that:

How these people are managed, what they are told, how they are told it and the accuracy of information that they are given is very important for the patients' subsequent management of herpes and their lives . . . It is almost negligent now not to offer oral treatment to those with a primary episode of genital herpes.

(Dayan 1994)

The 'Evian Declaration' which resulted from a meeting of physicians and people concerned about HSV recurrences sponsored by the American Social Health Association (ASHA) in 1992, discussed

issues related to the management of genital herpes and set down
'goals for improved future management of genital herpes' in the
form of 'consensus statement as guidelines for both providers and
receivers of care'. Acknowledging that:

> many individuals have often felt neglected by the medical profes-
> sion, whose role in the past has been mainly to treat the physical
> symptoms of the disease, with less regard for the total well-being
> and psyche of the affected individual.

The Declaration suggested that 'both the physical disease and the
psychosocial aspects of this disease are closely linked with the
natural evolution of the condition'.

From the shock of discovering that they have genital herpes to
the realization that this condition may recur, individuals with
genital herpes are subject to a vast array of emotions which cut
through to the most personal and intimate levels of existence,
with sometimes devastating consequences.

This 'template for care' was divided into 'psychosocial issues',
'medical issues', and 'shared management', and included the
improvement of doctors' understanding of 'the diagnosis and
management' of genital herpes, and the general public's understanding of the 'disease' in the hope of reducing the stigma
associated with it. Information-giving and counselling were recognised as important, and doctors advised to allow at least twenty
minutes at initial diagnosis for this. The following suggestions imply
an enormously increased input of health care resources, which some
would certainly consider over-kill and moving to the opposite
extreme from medical neglect:

- provide all affected individuals with adequate counselling and
  psychological support where necessary;
- teach individuals with genital herpes to recognize any warning
  signs of a recurrence of disease, and to seek immediate medical
  help;
- physician and patient should consider suppressive acyclovir
  therapy as a longer term management strategy, so that no patient
  experiences unnecessary distress or frequent recurrences.

DEALING WITH THE IMPACT AND GETTING ON WITH LIFE

If everybody with a recurrence of herpes simplex symptoms sought 'immediate medical help', the health service would be swamped with people seeking urgent medical intervention for a very common self-limiting condition. Most 'unnecessary distress' results from people's difficulties in dealing with the stigma associated with the condition. Accurate information and adequate counselling around the time of diagnosis, followed by access to self-help group support can make all the difference to a person's reaction and subsequent adjustment to having the condition. A study by Swanson and Chenitz (1993) found that the attitude of the health professional conveying the diagnosis significantly influenced the reactions of their informants: an attitude which was perceived as 'negative, uncaring or judgemental' exacerbated participants' upset, but:

> Health professionals who were perceived as concerned and empathic and who provided information and attempted to place herpes in a rational perspective were deemed helpful.

Swanson and Chenitz (1993) carried out a qualitative study using grounded theory and drawing on the work of Charmaz (1987) to describe 'the psychosocial process that young adults use in adapting to living with genital herpes'. Semi-structured interviews were conducted with seventy people between the ages of 18 and 35 years in the USA with recurrent genital symptoms of HSV. The data analysis resulted in the delineation of a process with three stages through which participants regained a valued sense of self 'within a society that shames persons with this disease'. The sociocultural meaning of the condition was clearly taken as an unquestioned assumption in this study. The first stage termed 'protecting oneself', involved 'guarding and defending against a tainted identity and a perceived sense of loss during the period of diagnosis'. The second stage of 'renewing oneself' 'involved taking action to reappraise the self by reaching out and striving to balance one's life' (see Chapter 3); and the third stage of 'preserving oneself' 'involved adopting a management style that allowed one to live with the disease in accordance with one's sense of self' (see Chapters 3 and 4).

The first phase of the overall process of adjustment described by Swanson and Chenitz (1993) was composed of the processes of 'attending', 'reacting', 'seeking explanations' and 'resisting loss'. As a result of attending to bodily symptoms and the need for care, study participants sooner or later received a diagnosis of herpes simplex infection. When the diagnosis was delayed this could result in frustration and dismay in the meantime. They found that study informants' responses to the diagnosis and its meaning ranged on a continuum from severe, or 'devastation', to much less severe, with the condition being seen as 'a common problem, not unlike having a cold'. The circumstances which would make it more likely that the reaction to diagnosis would be less severe were, they suggested: previous experience with having a chronic illness; suspecting that they had the condition so that the diagnosis did not come as a surprise; having a supportive partner; and a positive attitude on the part of the health professional who diagnosed them. The search for explanations often followed diagnosis, and was accompanied by feelings of betrayal and anger towards self and the supposed donor of the infection. Undoubtedly, as Swanson and Chenitz (1993) suggested, the process of seeking explanations was 'confounded' by the lack of awareness of most informants of the possibility of asymptomatic transmission, as well as the variability of symptom recurrence after infection.

The process of 'resisting loss' that Swanson and Chenitz describe as the fourth component of this initial process of adjustment to a diagnosis of HSV infection was 'the strategy used to withstand the interpretation of meaning of the disease in their lives'. They state that:

a diagnosis of genital herpes eroded self-esteem, raised suspicions of infidelity in a partner, lowered confidence in establishing close relationships, and threatened these young adults' sense of self . . . They feared that they were now different; they could not go back to their past lives; and their lives in the future would be constrained.

(Swanson and Chenitz 1993)

'The major consequence', these authors suggest, of the first stage of the process they describe, was a 'distancing of self from others to protect the self' because a 'devalued or tainted identity stigmatised them and acted as a barrier or potential barrier to intimacy and thus needed to be hidden from others'.

Concern about the implications of living with the condition and possible rejection by a future sexual partner, is a very common, almost inevitable aspect of coming to terms with the diagnosis. However, the situation described by Swanson and Chenitz, in which a highly negative and stigmatised meaning is attached to the condition and reinforced at diagnosis, causing a major reaction in terms of loss of self-esteem and impulse to go into hiding, is *not* inevitable. The personhood of an individual diagnosed with HSV infection need not be dominated and overwhelmed by the heap of negative labels which can be associated with 'herpes' so that they become nothing but a person with herpes. As these authors acknowledged, the way in which the condition is presented by the health professional making the diagnosis can be crucial. Access at an early stage to accurate information, support and counselling, whether from health professionals or knowledgeable self-help group members, can counteract the stigmatised image of the condition and influence positively an individuals' thoughts and feelings about living with HSV infection. This is likely to have a beneficial effect on how such individuals face the possible implications of the condition and learn to live with recurrences if they get them. 'Role engulfment' which involves 'the sudden or gradual collapse of the supports that uphold a person's conception of himself or herself as being socially acceptable' (Schur 1979: 243) is much less likely in these circumstances. Why and how this is so will be examined in subsequent chapters.

Chapter 3

Learning to live with HSV symptoms

Herpes simplex is a chronic condition which may express itself as intermittently recurring symptoms on the genitalia or around the mouth or (less often) elsewhere on the body, and learning to live with the virus may mean learning to live with recurrent outbreaks of symptoms. The nature of this problem, in physical terms, varies greatly. There is some evidence of this variation, though the samples surveyed are clearly biased towards the more problematic end of the continuum of people having HSV symptoms, since it is these people who are more likely to seek help of some sort from self-help groups or clinics. There are many more people with HSV who are never troubled by symptoms, either because the virus is dormant or because the symptoms are so mild they do not notice them, or so infrequent they are no problem. This chapter will review the experience of recurrences, and the important role of accurate information, empathic support and attitude change in the process of adapting to life with intermittent symptoms of HSV infection. The management strategies adopted as part of this process, experience of medical treatment and the evidence of benefit from 'psychosocial' interventions will be discussed. The final section of the chapter will review research studies of factors involved in positive adaptation and some personal accounts of the process.

THE RECURRENCE OF SYMPTOMS

A survey of 3,142 members of HELP (a national organisation in the USA for people with Herpes Simplex symptoms) found the median recurrent rates to be five to eight episodes per year (Knox et al. 1982). A 1988 membership survey of the UK Herpes Association (HA) (Posner 1990) found that nearly all 294 responding members experienced symptoms on the genitals, but some 12 per cent also had herpes simplex outbreaks around the mouth and 13 per cent also had symptoms elsewhere on the body. Most respondents (70 per cent) said they got herpetic symptoms in the genital area only. As can be seen in Table 3.1, the frequency of recurrences varied greatly: 22 per cent of respondents had symptoms more often than once a month, 15 per cent had them every month or almost every month, 23 per cent between five and eight times a year and 27 per cent between once and four times a year. Six per cent were no longer getting symptoms, and 7 per cent were uncertain about the frequency of recurrences. Mostly, the symptoms were experienced as moderate (41 per cent) or mild (37 per cent), but 17 per cent had found them severe.

Two years earlier a survey of its membership carried out by the HA itself (*Sphere*, 3(2)) had found a slightly different pattern of recurrences with roughly a third of respondents saying they had between one and four recurrences per year, a third between five and nine, and a third over ten. This questionnaire also asked if the recurrences were more often than the previous year. Nearly half (48 per cent) said they were the same, a third that they were less (33 per cent), and 19 per cent said they had increased. The researchers commented that since the medical prognosis is that herpes gets better over time, the fact that that this was not the case for a proportion of the membership sample 'must be to do with the fact that only people who are still getting a lot of attacks continue to belong to the HA for any length of time' (*Sphere*, 3(2): 17).

This survey also asked whether members had noticed a pattern to their recurrences, and what factors appeared to trigger them. Forty-five per cent of female and 46 per cent male members had perceived

Table 3.1 Frequency of HSV symptoms

	(N = 294) %
More than once a month	22
9-12 times a year	15
5-8 times a year	23
3-4 times a year	17
1-2 times a year	10
Not at all	6
Don't know/NA	7

Source: Herpes Association membership survey (Posner 1990)

a pattern. However, 43 per cent of respondents said that there was no pattern to their recurrences. The majority of respondents mentioned something they thought was a triggering factor. Stress was the most often mentioned (by 68 per cent) triggering factor, followed by menstruation for 40 per cent of the female respondents, and illness (mentioned by 27 per cent). An article in the HA's newsletter (*Sphere*, 8(3): 15) also mentioned stress, anxiety and depression, fatigue, menstruation, other infections such as colds and flu, and ultraviolet light as precipitating factors for recurrences, adding:

> However, in many patients, none of the above triggers will precipitate a recurrence, whilst they may have a recurrence for no apparent reason.

Both the predictability of recurrences in some cases and the unpredictability in others, causes distress. There are various sources of potential help for people who have to deal with recurrences of symptoms of HSV: their GP, GUM clinics, self-help organisations, women's health centres, books advising about self-care, and complementary practitioners. The role of the information and support provided by the HA (a national self-help organisation for people troubled by HSV in the UK), evidence of the range of individual management strategies, the use of medical treatment and the possible role of non-medical treatment, will be described. A helpful aspect of the condition not given much emphasis in the literature is that symptom recurrences will get better by themselves without any intervention of any kind. This means that however distressing in physical and/or psychological terms a particular recurrence may feel to the individual, experience over a period of time living with the condition will confirm the fact that it passes, life goes on, and it is not a significant threat to the individual's health in the longer term.

THE ROLE OF INFORMATION AND SUPPORT

In their conceptualisation of the process of adaptation to living with 'genital herpes' (discussed in Chapter 2), Swanson and Chenitz termed the second stage, 'Renewing Oneself'. This, they suggested involved seeking information, managing risks (particularly in relation to sexual relationships, discussed in Chapter 4) and balancing one's life.

> Seeking information consisted of finding resources in the community for information and for help in coping with the

disease. In this process, informants began to identify with others who had herpes.

(Swanson and Chenitz 1993)

Such information seeking might be carried out in low-risk activities such as listening to a telephone tape or reading relevant material in an anonymous setting such as a library, or it might involve taking the risk of admitting to having HSV infection, for instance to a counsellor or helpline volunteer. Through self-help organisations the individual would be in contact with 'veterans' who could take 'the role of coach or mentor'. The result of this information-seeking activity by the subjects of Swanson and Chenitz's study, was that:

Often, they became more knowledgeable about the disease than their health practitioners ... most informants learned what to expect in living with the disease and found out that others had similar experiences; this knowledge helped them to begin to deal with their loss and to gain the confidence to assess the risk of bringing up the subject with a partner.

(Swanson and Chenitz 1993)

In learning to live with this condition, the sources of information which HA members responding to the 1988 survey (Posner 1990) said they had found most useful were *Sphere* (the HA newsletter), mentioned by 68 per cent altogether, books, (the combination of *Sphere* and books was mentioned by 30 per cent), other group members, and the HA Helpline. There were some very negative comments about doctors in general, in this respect:

Most doctors are either indifferent or overbearingly moralistic.

Doctors have been *useless* – negative, condemning, or simply knew *nothing* about herpes at all and did not know of the HA.

However, there were also a few positive comments about the help-fulness of particular doctors and clinics.

HA members who had contacted the Helpline mentioned receiving information they found helpful and reassuring:

Marvellous to pick up the phone and find someone available and informed.

The HA is an invaluable source of information. Just knowing it's there is a great comfort.

Sometimes people contrasted this with their experience of medical services:

> I've found HA staff very helpful, friendly and have felt great sense of relief being able to turn to someone who is knowledgeable and trustworthy. I often found I'd learnt more about herpes than the doctors I was approaching, so when I was confused about something I trusted HA staff more than local doctors.

> I was amazed how little my local special clinic could do to help me come to terms with having herpes. The health adviser there was helpful later, but seemed to know little, and got most of her information from HA office via me.

> After phoning the Association, reading books and going to meetings, I found I knew more than my GP who received a copy of my notes. He now refers new patients to the HA.

The largest proportion (40 per cent) of comments on contact with the HA Helpline mentioned support received which was a facilitator of acceptance and adaptation to life with HSV through understanding and empathy, the breakdown of feelings of isolation, reassurance about various anxieties, and simply 'talking things through':

> At a time when I desperately needed help, it was the HA that was the first to help me come to terms with simplex.

> It was wonderful to be able to talk to someone who knew just what I was going through. It really helped to put things in perspective.

> Very caring response, reassuring and informative, a relief to discuss such personal matters with someone then unknown, in such an easy and open way.

> It [the Helpline] was the *only* place I could speak to anyone about it.

Letters written from the HA office were also mentioned by a few people as a form of contact they had appreciated and found helpful. An HA member's account of her personal experience (*Sphere*, 5(1): 12) is an illustration of the role such contact can play in changing a person's thinking and feelings about having HSV:

> I still felt as though I was the only one in the world with Simplex. I sank into bouts of depression, and desperately felt I needed

someone to talk to. I had so many feelings inside me. I felt unclean about myself and not like a woman, but, this 'female thing' with Simplex. I finally wrote a letter to the HA asking for help. I desperately needed support and the knowledge that I was not alone. Little did I know this would change my life . . . Having contact with others at the HA helped so much with coming to terms with Herpes Simplex and my feelings of low self worth. I now know a great deal depends on me and how I treat myself, feeling more in control of my life has been a great step for me and I now really believe I have the power to live a positive life with Simplex being a minor nuisance.

The reduction in isolation, depression and negative feelings, and the increase in self-esteem and self-efficacy described in this account, is the psychological and emotional accompaniment of the cognitive process involved in 'reframing'; together they provide fertile ground for positive adaptation to life with HSV symptom recurrences. Reframing is a term applied to the process of acknowledging the reality of an event but changing the way it is perceived, so that reactions to it also change. Swanson and Chenitz (1990) writing about health professional intervention in this process suggested:

The challenge . . . is how to increase patients' quality of life by reframing the image of the disease from negative to neutral and refocusing attention to self-care and adaptation.

This is something that many individuals can and will do for themselves as a result of becoming informed and their own experiential knowledge. Coming in contact with a view of the condition other than the stereotypical media 'hype' of the 1980s (as described in Chapter 1) is crucial to this process.

CHANGED VIEWS OF HSV

Insight into the elements of a changed perception of the condition has come from analysis of the answers to a question on the 1988 HA membership survey (Posner 1990) asking if respondents had learnt anything in particular about herpes simplex which had changed their view of the condition. Nearly two-thirds (61 per cent) replied that they had. For at least a quarter (26 per cent) this involved a changed view of the seriousness of the condition, expressed as:

I first thought herpes was a disaster, now I view it as a minor nuisance.

It's only the cold sore virus. This helps put it in perspective.

It is merely 'core sores' wherever it appears and is a minor skin condition rather than a syphilitic plague.

Realization that it is not a serious illness in that it does not incapacitate me and I can learn to live and cope with it.

The view that it is widespread and when considered unemotionally, a trifling complaint.

That it's a minor inconvenience which only visits occasionally, not a permanent affliction which never leaves.

To understand herpes in its true perspective rather than having the attitude that it is a devastatingly incurable disease, but just a minor problem.

The idea that herpes was 'not . . . a medically serious condition', in fact it can be so mild that people could have it without knowing that they were infected, and, in comparison with some other sexually transmitted conditions one could catch, such as syphilis or HIV, its medical consequences were minor, was a powerful one in transforming peoples' views.

There were many indications that respondents' original views of the condition had been strongly influenced by its presentation in the media, and information received from elsewhere had changed their thinking:

Knowing the facts – a relief after building up a picture of the illness from the press.

The only thing I first knew about herpes was that it was 'incurable'. Now I know how minor it is and I am infuriated when it is considered to be like AIDS (e.g. in the press).

I knew nothing about it until I caught it – I thought it was a lethal disease and put a stop to one's sex life for ever – all due to the media. Now I know about it, I realise this is all rubbish.

Not the great evil the media would have you believe – just a damned inconvenience.

This revision of view of the seriousness of the condition was an important aspect of the process of coming to terms with it, and getting it in perspective which respondents (24 per cent) wrote about, saying 'life is much the same after it', 'there's life after herpes' and 'it's not the end of the world'.

I have realised that it is only part of your life – something you have to live with and accept.

A fuller understanding – I can cope with it now.

Accepting things as they are and not letting it ruin my life.

Further analysis of the answers to this survey question revealed other things which had been learnt and found helpful in the process of acceptance and adaptation to life with recurrences of herpes simplex symptoms. The two most frequently mentioned were learning that many people have the condition (mentioned by 16 per cent), and that the condition is controllable or manageable (also mentioned by 16 per cent). In respect of the latter, various things were mentioned that could be done to help prevent recurrences (see 'Management strategies' below). As respondents explained:

Taking steps to control recurrences has made me feel less at the mercy of herpes.

If you stop worrying, and take care of yourself, you can reduce attacks.

Understanding the way the virus works and trying to control the number of outbreaks.

I do feel a lot of my problem is my attitude to having the virus, but the psychological difference of being able to do something about my attacks (control of diet/mental support from reading the newsletters has been enormous). I am doing something positive for myself.

Knowing that many 'other people have it and deal with it effectively' was further useful information in changing peoples' attitudes to HSV. For one thing it is 'reassuring to know you're not on your own' and are in good company:

Finding that herpes affects people from all walks of life, but they remain normal well-balanced beings.

Other people I like and respect also have herpes.

It can also be 'helpful to feel that other people face the same problems in their lives'. In particular, reading other's experiences helped counteract feelings of isolation and was encouraging:

A problem shared is a problem halved, once you realise that hundreds of people feel like you, you feel less isolated.

I feel less isolated and guilty now I have read and heard of other people's experiences – more 'normal'.

I found the condition is much more common than I thought and many people suffer recurrences. Consequently, I feel more confident about eventually controlling attacks at a manageable level, talking to prospective partners, and perhaps marriage.

A few people mentioned that they had come to the realisation that other people suffered more from recurrences than they did, and felt fortunate by comparison.

Feeling better about oneself, regaining one's sense of self-worth and identity, was an accompaniment of this revision of view of the condition, and an indicator of the process of coming to terms with having HSV, mentioned by 8 per cent of respondents:

I've stopped seeing myself as a 'leper' and just as someone who happens to have something to 'deal with' every now and then – I am still ME!

Reducing the stress of feeling like a leper. Helping myself feel normal and acceptable.

Herpes sufferers are not different from anyone else, e.g. a person who gets a lot of colds – that's a virus too. It's only taboo because it's on the genitals and it's sexually transmitted.

Feeling one could be an acceptable sexual partner was a very important aspect of this redefinition, and a few respondents mentioned that understanding and acceptance by a partner had been helpful. Respondents mentioned no longer feeling like a 'leper' or 'dirty':

One does not have to feel isolated or like a leper, or live a totally celibate life from reading *Sphere*.

It's not the end of any love life.

Learning that one was not constantly infectious, that transmission of the virus could be avoided, and that a sex life was still possible, was an important piece of information mentioned by 7 per cent of respondents, which clearly related both to their view of the virus and of themselves.

A similar number of people (7 per cent) indicated that the passage of 'time' had been helpful in altering their view of the condition:

The fact that it generally decreases in severity and frequency with time.

That it is normally a relatively harmless virus which over time becomes normally less and less of a problem.

The following answer encapsulates the process of acceptance of life with the herpes simplex virus over time:

Initial shock and depression. The Herpes Association and books and people helped; and time. Prefer not to have it, but now [it's] a 'monitor twitch' on my state of well being.

MANAGEMENT STRATEGIES

Acceptance of recurrences is part of the process of adjustment to living with symptoms of HSV infection. Finding a way to respond to recurrences in order to minimise physical discomfort or developing a strategy to try to avoid them altogether is another aspect of the adjustment process. The answers to a question on the 1988 HA membership survey (Posner 1990) inquiring if anything had been learnt which the respondent had found particularly helpful in dealing with recurrences, allowed the mapping of a large range of these sorts of responses and strategies. Just over half (56 per cent) the respondents noted something on the questionnaire. The answers to this question ranged from very general to highly specific approaches to managing recurrences. There were two types of general approach: *lifestyle* and *cognitive* (Table 3.2). The first was focused on maintaining a lifestyle which allowed one to reduce stress (mentioned in 24 per cent of answers), get enough sleep and rest (9 per cent), and look after one's general health (6 per cent).

Learning to relax and not worry, plenty of sleep – especially restricting hectic socialising – living a quieter, better balanced life, and maintaining a more positive attitude.

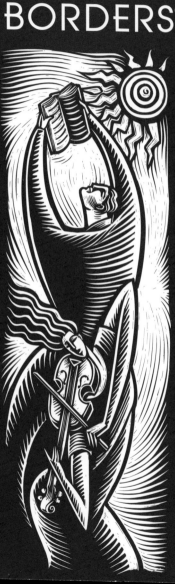

BORDERS®

30% OFF NEW YORK TIMES BESTSELLERS • 10% OFF MOST OTHER HARDCOVERS

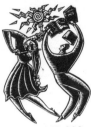

- over 150,000
  book titles

- over 60,000
  music titles

- over 8,000
  video titles

- 30% OFF
  New York Times &
  Chicago Tribune
  Hardcover Bestsellers

- 10% OFF
  most other
  hardcovers

- top 50 CD's and
  selected new releases
  specially priced
  every day

- special orders
  welcome

- free gift wrapping

- world-wide shipping

BORDERS®

830 N. Michigan Avenue
Chicago, IL 60611
(312)573-0564

Mon-Sat 8am-11pm
Sun 9am-9pm

Table 3.2 Elements of HSV symptom management strategies

			(% mentioning)
General approach			**60**
	Lifestyle:	reduce stress 24	
		sleep and rest 9	
		general health 6	
	Cognitive:	right attitude 15	
		understanding 6	
Diet			**41**
	General	15	
	Vitamins and	10	
	minerals		
	↑ L-lysine/	16	
	↓ L-arginine		
Medical/ pharmaceutical treatment			**35**
	Acyclovir	20	
	(Zovirax)		
	OTC medications	11	
	Complementary	4	
	therapies		
Topical treatment			**15**

Source: Herpes Association membership survey (Posner 1990)

As 'stress' especially of the emotional kind, seems to trigger an attack with me, I am trying to learn not to get into a state about things in general . . . unfortunately it's a bit of a vicious circle as I worry *mainly* about having herpes.

Lots of sleep. Don't let yourself get upset and run down.

Keeping mentally and physically fit and healthy to maintain a healthy immune system to help fight an attack.

The second was focused on having the right attitude (15 per cent) and involved understanding and information (6 per cent):

I feel recurrences are all in the mind. I have tried various remedies etc. but find the best one is simply to forget it or at least treat it as a minor irritation, rather like someone who suffers from say spots, athletes foot or mouth ulcers, etc.

I try not to concentrate too much on preventing recurrences as I feel that this almost allows the disease to take over one's life.

Suggestions involving diet included general dietary changes (mentioned in 15 per cent), and the adoption of a specific diet which involved increasing foods containing L-lysine and avoiding foods containing L-arginine (mentioned by 16 per cent):

> A dietary therapist . . . advised me to follow a vegan diet and to avoid wheat products, also to take a range of supplements (vitamins and minerals) with the aim of strengthening my immune system. This has improved my health in every way including reducing the severity of herpes attacks.

Taking additional vitamins and minerals, vitamin C and zinc in particular, was mentioned by 10 per cent of respondents. Altogether diet-related suggestions were mentioned in 41 per cent of answers to this question (Table 3.2).

Some form of medical or pharmaceutical treatment was mentioned in 31 per cent of answers: acyclovir (Zovirax) ointment or tablets were mentioned most frequently (20 per cent) (Table 3.2). A smaller proportion of answers (11 per cent) mentioned over-the-counter (OTC) medications or other treatment: antibiotic or antiseptic cream or powder (Betadine, Cicatrin, Dermatabs), aspirin, and 'Dr Skinner's vaccine'. Various forms of complementary medical approaches such as hypnosis, self-hypnosis and homeopathy were mentioned by relatively few respondents (4 per cent of answers).

Topical treatment of sores was a feature of 15 per cent of the answers (Table 3.2), with taking salt baths mentioned most often. The various other means of drying or soothing the sores mentioned were surgical spirit (only for the hardy), witch hazel, ice cubes, cold wet cotton wool, and using a blow dryer.

As with other conditions subject to symptomatic variations and not very amenable to medical control, such as multiple sclerosis (Robinson 1988) or chronic fatigue syndrome (CFS), people with the condition devise their own idiosyncratic control stratagems, adding various components together. These are some examples:

> Emphasis on one, diet, two, exercise and stress reduction; and realisation that I need to try to ignore the thing while trying to live, to reduce its impact on me.

> Yoga. Meditation. Self-hypnosis. Sleep.

> Vitamin C. No stress. No chocolate/nuts. Healthy diet.

Good night's sleep. Orange juice (vitamin C). Keep relaxed and not to worry about problems. Sports and good diet (onion will help), fresh fruit, brown bread, all bring less attacks.

Beyond these management strategies, and interweaving the different components, some people held theories about controlling the condition:

I have 'Zovirax' and would take drugs, but prefer a 'natural health' approach. Recurrences happen, I believe, due to less than healthy immune system – which is affected psycho-physically by external factors (stress: job, relationships, weather, etc., etc.) and internal factors (stress: reactions, mind). Diet: I avoid arginine foods and go for lysine rich foods – an important factor. Physical well being: especially Tai Chi which gently improves the immune system.

Information on dealing with stress and how that makes the immune system less able to cope with the virus and makes you prone to attacks. I've taken more vitamins and avoided stress, etc., i.e. taken steps by myself which made me feel more in control and in turn have helped me cope and not feel so over-whelmed. Learning acyclovir tablets are available has helped at times when I couldn't cope with another attack, though I wouldn't want to take it long term.

The HA's newsletter regularly informs its readers about possible treatments: medical developments and research trials, as well as complementary therapies such as homeopathic remedies, hypnotherapy, dietary intervention on the basis of the lysine/arginine theory (*Sphere*, 2(7)). In 1993/4, ninety-three volunteer HA members took part in a six-month double-blind placebo-controlled trial of 'Elagen' – the trade name for the standardised form of the herbal medicine Eleutherococcus senticosus (ES) – which the organisation helped administer. The results indicated that subjects taking Elagen had 'shorter, fewer and less severe outbreaks' (*Sphere*, 9(3): 5).

RESEARCH STUDIES OF PSYCHOSOCIAL INTERVENTIONS

There have been a number of reports of studies of non-medical interventions with individuals troubled by herpes simplex recurrences.

The study by Blank and Brody (1950) of psychoanalytically-oriented, suggestive therapy was probably the first. Several therapists have used a combination of hypnosis with other interventions such as cognitive restructuring, self-hypnosis or supportive psychotherapy. The efficacy of progressive muscle relaxation training has been studied by VanderPlate and Kerrick (1985) and Burnette et al. (1991). McLarnon and Kaloupek (1988) compared randomly assigned cognitive restructuring and structured discussion treatments in terms of symptom recurrence frequency, psychological distress, and coping. Five small group sessions were held for each treatment condition in which the participants discussed their initial reactions to acquiring the infection, their difficulties talking to others including potential sexual partners about it, and the effect of the condition upon them. The cognitive restructuring group were given exercises and homework assignments in addition. Participants of this group experienced significant decreases in recurrence rates between post treatment and the twelve-week follow-up when compared to the structured discussion group; but neither group experienced significant reductions in distress or loneliness. These studies involved small numbers, lacked control groups, mostly did not have baseline measurements, involved self-reports of recurrences and did not have long-term follow-up measurements (and thus did not control for the intermittency of HSV symptoms).

An investigation by Longo, Clum and Yaeger (1988) which did involve a control group, prospective monitoring and clinical verification of HSV symptoms throughout the study, randomly allocated thirty-one patients to one of three groups: psychosocial treatment, social support or waiting list control. Again, the treatment was conducted in small groups across six sessions. The psychosocial intervention included information on HSV, sharing feelings, stress management, relaxation and imagery techniques. Participants in the social support group had the opportunity to discuss their feelings and interpersonal experiences related to having herpes simplex recurrences. Standardised measures of psychological variables were used. The psychosocial intervention resulted in greater improvement in emotional distress, mood, loneliness and health locus of control, as well as significantly fewer recurrences of HSV symptoms, than either the social support group or the waiting list condition.

The benefits reported by members of therapy groups have also been reported, as described previously, by people in contact with a self-help group for people troubled by HSV diagnosis or recurrences, and by some, though not all, participants in the meetings of support groups (Chapter 4). How beneficial such contact will be, is likely to depend on the interpersonal skills of the contact persons, and in groups, on how difficult issues and negativity is handled. Some individuals may need one-to-one counselling, particularly in the early stages of learning to live with recurrences of HSV symptoms. In their review of psychosocial factors in recurrent genital symptoms of HSV, Longo and Koehn (1993) concluded:

> Psychological treatments are superior to supportive interventions and/or no treatment. The combined results of these studies suggest that while providing HSV information, social support, and discussions of herpes related concerns is beneficial for many herpes sufferers, treatments that incorporate specific coping methods are superior to mere supportive psychotherapy. Furthermore, therapeutic interventions which include relaxation-based training, stress management, and cognitive restructuring skills, appear to provide the greatest gains for individuals with recurrent genital herpes.

Effective self-help organisations and support groups may provide in a less structured way and for larger numbers what therapy groups and individual therapy provide for a few.

MEDICAL TREATMENT

Medical treatment for HSV recurrences has been largely confined to acyclovir (brand name, Zovirax) either in the form of cream or tablets, which was introduced in the early 1980s (Chapter 1). The use of this drug has increased considerably since then, reflecting increasing recognition of psychosocial distress caused by HSV recurrences and Wellcome's promotion of its product. The HA's own surveys of its membership (*Sphere*, 2(7), 7(4)) asking about the availability, use and effectiveness of acyclovir in 1986 and 1992 showed the use of acyclovir increased between the first and second survey. The proportion of the membership responding to the questionnaires was relatively low both times, 42 per cent and nearly 30 per cent respectively, but is likely to have been drawn from those more troubled by symptoms and more likely to be using medication. Nearly everyone had heard of acyclovir, mostly from medical sources or the HA, but also from newspapers, magazines and books, and occasionally from friends.

In 1986, 76 per cent of respondents had used acyclovir, predominantly for genital symptoms, and mostly regularly, with each recurrence (65 per cent). The largest group in the sample (36 per cent) used the cream alone, 30 per cent used the cream and tablets, and 10 per cent the tablets alone to treat recurrences. Only a small proportion were taking the tablets continuously at that date. In 1992, 83 per cent of the survey responders had used acyclovir, again mostly for genital HSV infection (though between 7 per cent and 8 per cent used it for facial symptoms as well), 54 per cent were using acyclovir for each recurrence, using either the cream only (59 per cent), or tablets only (27 per cent) or both (14 per cent). Altogether 83 per cent of the sample had used acyclovir cream, 70 per cent had used the tablets and 53 per cent had used both. There was clearly a large increase in the proportion taking acyclovir tablets. At this date, at least 16 per cent were taking tablets as suppressive therapy.

The HA's surveys found that in 1986, 13 per cent, and in 1992, 19 per cent reported side effects that respondents attributed to acyclovir. In 1992, nearly a quarter (24 per cent) of the survey sample felt that acyclovir was useful for treating recurrences because it reduced symptoms. Among those using either tablets or cream to treat each recurrence, a considerably higher proportion thought tablets 'stopped' or 'decreased the number' of recurrences. Among those using tablets for suppressive treatment, 78 per cent of men and 73 per cent of women had found that it was effective in stopping recurrences. There appeared to be a drop in the proportion (from 33 per cent to 7 per cent) who thought that acyclovir was no help at all, probably related to the increase in tablet takers.

The second HA survey investigated the instructions respondents reported being given about the use of acyclovir tablets and cream and found very considerable variations, many not in accord with the pharmaceutical company's directions. Among those prescribed acyclovir tablets for their primary episode (first occurrence of symptoms associated with initial infection), only 26 per cent of male members and 32 per cent of female members appeared to have been given the correct instructions. Among those prescribed acyclovir cream, 61 per cent of the male members and 48 per cent of the female members said they were given no instructions. The HA report of the survey findings expressed concern that so many women with genital symptoms had been prescribed the cream rather than tablets, despite the fact that the medication is not recommended for the vaginal mucous membrane because it can cause irritation and maceration. (Nine per cent of women using the cream complained of associated irritation and discomfort). The cream is suitable for dry skin areas only, but genital symptoms in women are often around the membranous area.

Survey responders reported some reluctance and outright refusals to prescribe acyclovir, mostly on the grounds of cost. In 1992, 18 per cent (two-thirds of whom were male) had been refused a prescription at some time; in 1986, 14 per cent (males and females equally) had reported a refusal. Certainly, acyclovir is comparatively expensive, and this is a factor to take into account in opting for suppressive treatment. However, this unusual concern with the cost of prescriptions (largely pre-dating GP budget-holding) may also have reflected an attitude that patients with HSV do not deserve or do not really need relief from the symptoms. It is noteworthy that, according to this HA survey, doctors appear to be more willing to supply acyclovir to women than men. Nearly half (47 per cent) the male responders and a third of the female responders were not prescribed acyclovir during their primary HSV episode. Twice as many men (44 per cent) as women (22 per cent) were not offered treatment at any time. There is some evidence that females have slightly more severe symptoms in terms of pain and the time taken to heal (*Medical Observer*, 14 May 1993: 12). Whether GPs took account of this in their decisions to prescribe or withhold acyclovir is not clear.

According to an investigation of the views of 112 GUM consultants in the UK carried out by the HA, the main reason for prescribing acyclovir as suppressive treatment is 'to decrease psychological morbidity' and the prime factors influencing a prescription are the patients being 'very anxious' or 'stressed/run down' (personal communication). Do female patients more convincingly express their anxiety, stress and psychological distress, or are they more readily 'allowed' to be in such a state? The 1992 HA survey also asked about the attitudes of members' GPs to their condition and found that a higher proportion of women (45 per cent) than men (33 per cent) considered their GP to be sympathetic rather than indifferent (37 per cent of women, 49 per cent of men) or moralistic (6 per cent of women, 8 per cent of men). When asked about their GP's knowledge of HSV, 59 per cent thought it very good or adequate, whereas 79 per cent thought the GUM clinic doctors' knowledge was very good or adequate. One female respondent reported that her GP told her she had thrush when she was 'bed-ridden, unable to walk and covered in sores' (*Sphere*, 7(4): 11). There were a number of reported instances of female patients being told they had thrush rather than herpes simplex.

In a letter to the *Lancet*, Mindel (1990) questioned the frequent reluctance on the part of GPs and genitourinary physicians to prescribe acyclovir for recurrent genital symptoms of HSV, suggesting that 'the introduction of suppressive oral acyclovir had revolutionised the treatment of this condition', and that most patients on treatment had no recurrences or only minor outbreaks, were less depressed about their condition and 'able to have normal sexual relations'. It was his practice to consider all patients with frequently recurring genital herpes for treatment, and he argued that the cost of the drug was not a justification for withholding treatment.

POSITIVE ADAPTATION

'Balancing One's Life' was the final phase of the second ('Renewing Oneself') stage of the process of adapting to life with recurrences of herpes simplex mapped by Swanson and Chenitz (1993). This phase involved managing symptoms, possible life-style changes and refocusing on other things in life besides HSV infection. A positive consequence of this stage of successful adaptation, they suggested, was 'reaffirmation of self'. However, when an individual does not get helpful information and has unsatisfactory interpersonal interactions, positive affirmation of the self is not likely to occur. 'These informants became more isolated, avoided social activities, and were often left without support and the confidence to tell others', Swanson and Chenitz (1993) reported.

There have been a number of attempts to investigate the psychosocial factors associated with positive adaptation, indicators of psychological adjustment or ways of coping, in relation to recurrences of herpes simplex symptoms in the genital area. Keller, Jadack and Mims (1991) examined coping responses, as indicated by the Coping Orientations to Problems Experienced (COPE) Scale (Carver, Scheier and Weintraub 1989) in relation to four of the 'most upsetting stressors' identified by the sixty subjects in their study. Study participants reported using a wide variety of coping responses, but individuals appeared to cope in a similar manner with each of four consequence-related stressors. 'Acceptance' ('accepting the reality of a situation') was the most frequent coping response, 'planning' ('active development of a plan to best handle the situation') and 'restraint' ('waiting for an appropriate opportunity to act') were also frequently reported coping mechanisms. Keller et al. suggested that this finding indicated that their subjects were 'actively trying to resolve problems associated with the disease'.

Manne and Sandler (1984) looked at coping mechanisms and their correlation with measures of psychological adjustment in 152 subjects who were members of self-help groups and volunteer participants. Stress thoughts concerning herpes simplex were the strongest predictor of overall adjustment and accounted for 39 per cent of the variance. Length of time since infection and severity of symptoms accounted for only an additional 1.8 per cent of the variance. There was a negative correlation between being depressed or being bothered by herpes simplex, and the length of time a subject had had HSV infection. Higher levels of social support were correlated with less symptomatology and higher self-esteem. The perceived helpfulness of support was correlated with better overall adjustment and fewer sexual problems. Study participants who perceived the attitude of family friends and health workers as more negative, reported a greater degree of depression, more sexual problems, poorer self-esteem, and poorer overall adjustment. Against expectations, problem-focused coping and minimisation of threat (represented by HSV infection) were not significantly correlated with any of the adjustment measures. Greater use of disease management strategies was significantly correlated with depression but not highly correlated with overall adjustment.

The study reported above tried to unravel the complex interrelationships between psychological variables and various indicators of successful adjustment. It confirmed the association between negative cognitions and poor adjustment (and thus the importance of how herpes simplex infection is presented and thought about, in relation to experience of the condition), and the benefit, in various ways, of social support. This is in line with the evidence from the survey of the UK Herpes Association members presented earlier in this chapter. As Manne and Sandler (1984) noted, 'negative cognitions are potentially manipulatable variables'. One way informants quoted earlier in this chapter reported that this happened was through minimisation of the threat represented by HSV infection:

for instance when it was understood that the condition was very common and not a major threat to health or child-bearing. However, Manne and Sandler's study could not confirm the benefit of minimisation of the seriousness of herpes simplex in terms of the adjustment variables measured. The implied usefulness (psychologically and/or physically) of the variety of management strategies reported by Herpes Association informants was also not reflected in this study's finding that the *number* of disease management strategies employed was associated with higher depression scores. These authors' interpretation of this finding was that it was related to psychopathology because it indicated obsession, a lack of acceptance of the situation, and use of a coping mechanism unlikely to resolve the 'stressor', and they suggested that:

> The attempts to gain control of herpes, and the repeated failures to do so, may lead to increased feelings of stress, helplessness and depression.
>
> (Manne and Sandler 1984)

It is likely that the 'disease management strategies' scale which included the use of self-initiated strategies to improve general health (and involving internal locus of control), as well as the numbers of visits to doctors and clinics (involving external locus of control), was not sufficiently discriminating, and was measuring different aspects of engagement with the condition. Manne and Sandler (1984) concluded that their study had shown coping mechanisms were better predictors of psychological variables than were the physical symptoms associated with HSV recurrences.

One of the subscales on the COPE Scale is termed 'Positive reinterpretation and growth' and was found by Keller, Jadack and Mims (1991) to be a frequently-used response to stressors related to living with HSV symptom recurrences. This response was reflected in the reframing which resulted in the changed views of HSV discussed above and in reports of other changes resulting from the process of coming to terms with life with herpes simplex. Accounts of people's attempts to adapt to life with an illness or chronic condition very often include a recognition of positive benefits resulting from the attitudinal or other changes made. So, too, with recurrent symptoms of herpes simplex, which can lead to taking stock of life, including a re-examination of values and priorities, and paying more attention to one's health. Sue Blanks, one of the founders of the HA, wrote in an article in *Woman* (16 April 1993) that for her:

Coming to terms with herpes is a long business but a lot of good can come out of it. It's made me examine my values, the way I live my life and what's important about me and about other people.

As with other threats to a person's health or well-being, facing the possible implications of a diagnosis of HSV infection, or the effects on the individual life of symptom recurrence, may involve a process of personal growth. Because of their testaments, we know that for some individuals herpes simplex has played a crucial role in their personal journeys. One author wrote about the way she had changed in the four years since she had been diagnosed with HSV infection (*Sphere*, 9(3): 12):

> I think I have changed quite a lot as a person. I think I now have a broader and more open view on a lot of things and that's a change in myself that I like.

This author suggested that she might not have grown or developed as a person in the same way or as much if she had not been through the experience:

> It's through the painful times that you begin to learn more about yourself as a person, although when you *are* suffering, that's probably the last thing on your mind.

Explaining that HSV had been a 'catalyst' which had caused her to examine her 'values, hopes, dreams and sense of self', another author (*Sphere*, 8(4): 11) listed a whole range of changes she had made in her 'long hard battle to reach . . . acceptance and peace'. These changes included stepping up her intake of multi-vitamins and minerals, eating more healthily, trying to sleep enough, using a homeopathic remedy and aromatherapy, and becoming a Christian and developing a spiritual life which enabled her to find 'great reserves of peace, joy and strength' within herself.

In the accounts of their personal experiences of coming to terms with HSV in the HA's newsletter, a number of authors wrote of what the condition had contributed to their lives 'along the road to recovery and acceptance', as one author put it (*Sphere*, 5(3): 12), rather than taken away, and how it had led to changes which they viewed as beneficial, such as being a 'stronger' person.

> It's been a long journey with herpes, but it's made me so much stronger personally now and I'm not afraid to love or feel guilty

about making love and know it really is O.K. to have herpes . . .
Herpes isn't just negative. Because of what I've been through, I'm
now more understanding of other people who may be in pain.
Sometimes you're given the bad things to see the good things.

(*Sphere*, 3(3): 11)

It's having herpes that changed my life for the better . . . I cannot
put into words *how much* simplex has done for me . . . I used to
take my health for granted . . . herpes simplex helped me focus
on what I *had*. And our health is the most precious gift of all.

(*Sphere*, 9(1): 8)

The next chapter will examine the area of social relations, which
is perhaps the most crucial forum for successful adaptation to life
with recurrent symptoms of herpes simplex.

Chapter 4

Social implications

There is much evidence that the problematic aspect of having herpes simplex for many people is psychosocial rather than physical or medical, and results from a fracturing of self-perceptions and social lives. The person troubled by HSV symptom recurrences has to deal not only with their own but also with others' feelings and thoughts about the condition. This would be the case with any chronic condition, but where a condition is stigmatised and transmissible, it poses additional problems of adaptation for the individual in terms of preserving a sense of an acceptable self. Learning to live with symptoms of HSV infection in the genital area entails negotiation of acceptance in certain social, particularly sexual, contexts, and the management of risk – the risk of rejection and the risk of transmission (Swanson and Chenitz 1993). This chapter will examine the social implications of life with recurrent genital symptoms, focusing on understandings of stigma, perceptions of handicap in personal relations, meeting others living with herpes simplex in groups and the negotiation of sexual relationships.

STIGMA

The cultural context from which the stigma associated with 'herpes' has arisen, was discussed earlier. The stigma has elements of both achievement and ascription: part of the shame results from the sexually transmitted nature of the condition, related to the person's own actions; however, there is a particular shame associated with 'genital herpes' which is not associated with genital warts for instance, though warts might be acquired from the same actions. The attached stigma carries implications both about the nature of the condition and about the nature of the person with the condition: the condition is shameful and the person known to have it, is judged essentially imperfect with a 'spoiled identity' (Goffman 1963).

In accepting that the condition of recurrent herpes simplex is part of their life, individuals who are aware of the stigma will need to find some way of adapting to its implications for their identity and social relations. In terms of their personhood, their response may be anything from totally accepting the stigmatising implications as truth about their value as persons, with a consequently catastrophic loss of self-esteem, to completely dismissing the implications as nothing to do with them as individuals. Since the genital symptoms of the condition are invisible in usual social circumstances, and the oral symptoms do not carry the same stigma (although they may *be* the same condition, as we have seen), people suffering from the condition will only need to negotiate its stigmatising implications socially in situations of sexual intimacy or potential intimacy. The individual could choose to avoid such situations altogether, and this is one form of adjustment. In this way they will be potentially 'discreditable' but avoid being 'discredited' (Goffman 1963). They will be acting in this way because of the 'felt' stigma, the shame they feel, but they will not suffer 'enacted' stigma, actual discrimination, because of it. They will avoid the pain of possible rejection and loss of another's esteem if they keep it secret in this way. However, the avoidance of sexual intimacy, if this means the absence of a close personal relationship or partnership, is a highly significant deprivation. This means that the focus of the stigma associated with this condition is in a very important area of life as far as most people are concerned. This is the core of the psychosocial problem of herpes simplex infection in the genital area.

In analysing ways of adapting to another stigmatised condition, epilepsy, Schneider and Conrad (1981) suggested three types of 'adjusted adaptation'. The 'pragmatic' type involves making light of the condition, not telling people about it indiscriminately because of the possibility of negative judgements, but on a 'need to know' basis, and in this way trying to minimise the impact of the condition. The 'secret' type of adaptation involves going to whatever lengths are necessary to conceal information about the stigmatised condition. These lengths may include lying on official forms. The 'quasi-liberated' type involves deliberately broadcasting the condition in an attempt to undermine the stigma and 'free one's self of the burdens of secrecy and concealment based on fear of stigma' (Schneider and Conrad 1981: 216). In other words, this form of adaptation is openly challenging the values and norms which attach discreditable meanings to the physical condition. Adjusted types of adaptation allow the person effectively to neutralise the actual or perceived negative impact of the stigmatised condition on their lives. Where the impact of the condition and its stigma is not managed in any kind of controlled way, as in the above strategies, the 'unadjusted' type of adaptation results in a person's identity being submerged by the negative connotations. In an extreme case this produces a 'debilitated' type of response in which an individual 'embraces epilepsy as an indelible and irrevocable threat to one's worth' (Schneider and Conrad 1981: 217). In these cases, the stigma becomes a 'master status' in which the person's whole identity and approach to life is determined by meanings and behaviour associated with that status, rather than any of the other statuses she or he may have. This is parallel to the concept of 'role engulfment' outlined by Schur (1979: 243). People diagnosed with HSV may have this kind of reaction, which may be a step on their path to a more positive permanent adjustment:

> Although I read many encouraging articles about Sex after Herpes, I buried myself away for six months – really did feel like a leper and didn't want to mix socially for I felt that there was no point as there was something so badly wrong with me.
>
> (*Sphere*, 2(7): 12)

Thus, as Scambler (1984: 218) wrote about epilepsy, 'felt stigma' may exact 'a considerable toll'.

In their conceptualisation of the process of adjustment to life with HSV recurrences, based on a qualitative study of young adults, Swanson and Chenitz (1993) suggested the final stage entailed 'preserving oneself'. Crucial to this preservation was the management of information about oneself in such a way that it enabled the individual to live with the condition and have an acceptable sense of self. They found three main styles of controlling information about the condition: 'accommodating' in which disclosure was conditional, 'avoiding' which was adopted by those who thought of themselves as having a 'permanent flaw', and 'revealing' in which disclosure was routine. These styles are clearly similar with the 'pragmatic', 'secret' and 'quasi-liberated' types of adaptation described by Schneider and Conrad (1981).

One way of trying to deal with the stigma attached to 'herpes' is not to use that name. This immediately loosens the association, allowing it to be questioned or shifted. For a period, the UK Herpes Association (HA) attempted to do this by referring to the condition as 'simplex'. This has a parallel in the terminology applied to another herpetic condition (herpes zoster), popularly known as 'shingles', and often referred to as 'zoster'.

I now˘chose to call the problem *'Simplex'*, for me not only a more medically accurate term, but also one which is free of publicity drenched 'hype' and reduces the condition to a more realistic level. It is simple.

(Workshop attendee reported in *Sphere*, 9(2): 12)

The HA has broadened its focus in recent years providing a service also to people with post-herpetic neuralgia following an episode of herpes zoster. At the end of 1994, a decision was taken to change the name of the association from simply 'Herpes . . . ' to either the 'Herpes *Simplex* Association' or the 'Herpes *Viruses* Association'. The name 'Herpes Viruses Association' was chosen and thus the possible membership now includes those with non-stigmatised human herpes viruses such as chicken pox, glandular fever and shingles.

PERCEPTION OF HANDICAP

A question in a membership survey of the HA (Posner 1990) asked if 'having herpes [was] a handicap in personal relationships'. There was a mixed response with a large majority acknowledging that it could be a handicap: 38 per cent thought it was definitely a handicap; nearly half (49 per cent) that it could be; and 12 per cent that it was not really a handicap. Where it was felt *not* to be a problem, this was, for the most part, because of steady relationships with partners who were accepting and understanding, or because symptoms were non-existent or infrequent, or because it was viewed as an inconvenience which can be circumvented rather than a disability. Where it *was* seen as a problem in personal relationships, this was because of the possibility of rejection by potential sexual partners or because of anxiety about passing it on, which made one respondent feel 'an outcast', another 'unable to participate' (in personal relationships), and because it could be a 'cause of stress in a sexual relationship which doesn't go away'. Many respondents qualified their answer by saying that whether it was a handicap depended on the attitude, knowledge and understanding of other people, or the sufferer's own attitude or feelings, and the context, specifically, whether it was social or sexual.

The social nature of the perceived handicap expressed in people's accounts of their attempts to come to terms with the condition, is reiterated time and again in descriptions of feelings of being isolated with and by a stigmatised and secret condition.

> I think the feeling of isolation herpes can give you is far more detrimental than any physical effects it has.
>
> (*Sphere*, 6(1): 8)

It was the social unacceptability of the condition which was so isolating. Describing the impact of the presentation of herpes in the media at a time when he was vulnerable, one sufferer described how he 'retracted back into my shell, cringing'. Another explained how herpes had made a radical difference in her or his life, saying:

> Herpes was a catalyst – I was a gregarious, outgoing, talkative person; I'm now the opposite.

Nearly all the sample of ten HA group members interviewed by the author, gave social contact as their main reason for joining the association. They wanted the opportunity to meet other people with the same condition because of the need they felt to talk about having herpes simplex and to 'unburden' themselves of something felt to be a stigma which was hidden in most social situations. One interviewee said:

> I just felt I had a terrible secret and I didn't want to be walking about with a terrible secret.

A second interviewee referred to it as 'the deepest, darkest secret' which she had kept for a long time. With the hidden stigma acknowledged and accepted, because it was shared by the other members of the group, it was possible to feel a sense of normality again:

> The one place one can be and you can feel quite normal.

Part of this normality was feeling acceptable to members of the opposite sex.. 'I thought I couldn't talk to a woman again', one HA group member interviewed explained. In answer to a question asking in what ways group members could help each other, two interviewees mentioned how talking to others with the condition broke down the feelings of social isolation:

> By talking about it . . . to help break this dreadful circle: having it makes you introverted – stops you going out – and this makes you more introverted.

> Just being able to talk about it because it isolates people – you can mention what is basically taboo.

The perception that having herpes simplex was a possible handicap in personal relationships was clearly an important motivator for joining the HA and going to group meetings. Responses to questions in the interviews conducted with HA support group members demonstrate elements of the handicap. In answer to a question asking if having herpes 'had made a lot of difference' in their life, all except one person said it had, and seven people talked in terms of the social implications, six mentioning the effect on sexual relationships. One person, who had become celibate, said that it was 'the most important thing that happened' to him in his twenties, that it had 'affected him profoundly'. Another respondent said that the condition had resulted in 'clinging to relationships' which s/he would have left earlier otherwise. Four group members spoke of hesitancy about potential sexual relationships: because of 'fear of scaring the person off', or because of avoidance of casual relationships. Another interviewee said that it had reduced her sex life, because 'it's made contact with men extremely difficult'. Asked if the condition was 'interfering with [their] life in any way now', nearly half the sample (4/10) spoke of the effect on (sexual) relationships:

> [It's] the whole basis of getting into a relationship.

> Only in terms of relationships. You just need to get your attitude right.

> Sexually – when I have it.

> Inhibits contacts with men.

MEETING OTHERS IN GROUPS

About half this sample of group members said their attitude to having the condition had changed and they had been 'helped to cope more easily with any aspect of having herpes' as a result of attending meetings or social events. In many cases, these attitude changes and ways of coping had implications for relationships.

I feel better about it – less hung up about it – less guilty – better equipped to cope with the next relationship – less like an outcast.

I like talking to people who cope with it well. It's some terrible social–sexual stigma. I'm still very touchy about it – feel very vulnerable about it. I would pay hundreds of pounds to get rid of it.

It's made me realise that anyone can have it – different ages, classes. The most helpful thing is meeting men.

Having met normal people – I'm not a social outcast any more. I feel more natural with women now.

Over half (58 per cent) the members responding to an HA membership survey (Posner 1990) had never been to a group meeting, and of these members, 42 per cent thought they did not know anyone else with herpes simplex. Among the survey responders who had at one time been to a group meeting, 45 per cent said that they had been only once, 29 per cent that they had been 'sometimes', and only 12 per cent that they had attended regularly. Contact with other people with the same condition can help in coming to terms with living with it by reducing feelings of isolation and increasing confidence that it is possible to lead a normal life.

For most HA survey responders who had been to a group meeting, the best thing about going, put simply, was the opportunity for identification with others with the same predicament, for sharing and for solidarity. Finding that other people with the condition were 'normal and decent', 'human and ordinary' and being able to identify with them was seen as an important benefit of going to a group by 38 per cent of members (Table 4.1). It means that 'you're not alone or even strange', 'that you are not a leper'. Being with other people with herpes simplex recurrences allowed some members to feel more at ease socially because they did not need to feel that they were 'the only one with HSV and therefore different', nor that they had 'a nasty secret hidden from them'.

Gaining or exchange of information was mentioned by 20 per cent; sharing experiences, concerns, anxieties, feelings and opinions with 'sympathetic people who know what you are talking about', by 30 per cent (Table 4.1). Sharing in this way, helped to 'reduce

Table 4.1 Benefits of group meetings

	(% mentioning)
Meeting other people with herpes simplex	38
Getting information	20
Sharing experiences and concerns	30
Mutual support and understanding	25
Helping others with herpes simplex	5

Source: Herpes Association membership survey (Posner 1990)

bitterness', 'put things in perspective' and 'laugh about it'. In particular, the opportunity to 'talk openly' and 'without fear or shame' with people 'one can be totally honest with about the condition' was seen as valuable. Being in a group with other members, provided, as one member wrote:

A chance to talk to people with similar problems in a way that would be difficult with non-sufferers.

The feelings of togetherness and reassurance, mutual support and understanding, kindness and caring, which resulted from being able to meet, talk and identify with others in this way, were seen as one of the best things about group meetings by 25 per cent (Table 4.1). One member expressed the reassurance s/he received as 'help with the initial gloom, doom and end-for-ever-of-any-sex feeling'. Members went not only to receive, but also to give reassurance, support and help to others, and in particular to those who had recently joined the group, and 5 per cent mentioned this (Table 4.1).

In this HA membership survey (Posner 1990) members were asked if there was anything which 'put them off going to a group meeting'. A quarter of responders mentioned practical difficulties such as inconvenient meeting times, or the difficulty of getting to the nearest group because of the distance or expense of travel, or lack of transport. Fifteen per cent were hesitant to go to a group because of shyness, nervousness, lack of confidence and anxieties about what the group would be like. A small percentage (7 per cent) said that shame or embarrassment put them off going to a meeting. Being able to speak to someone on the phone and meet that person beforehand can be helpful in easing a new member's introduction to a group.

While it was acknowledged that new members in particular, might be helped by meeting others at a group meeting, some responders indicated that they were at a different stage in the trajectory of their acceptance of life with HSV. Ten per cent felt that they no longer needed the group because they had support from people close to them, because the condition was no longer a problem, or because they had come to terms with it. Beyond this, there was the suggestion that continuing to go to a group could be unhelpful – as one member wrote, 'a reminder of what I've left behind'. Nine per cent said that they had been put off going to group meetings because of negative aspects of the interaction, finding it depressing to 'rehash . . . painful feelings relating to herpes' and to see others 'so miserable and despairing', 'despondent', 'vociferous and pessimistic', 'worried and upset'. A member who expressed this reason very clearly for not going to group meetings, wrote:

> I didn't really find the meetings that helpful as I had really come to terms with my herpes already, and meeting people who were still so 'screwed up' over it made me feel worse again and I started to get depressed and *think* about my condition and feel angry with life.

Furthermore, attending a group was seen by some (13 per cent) as working counter to the way in which they had dealt with having HSV, and suggested that concentrating or dwelling on it, talking or thinking about it, could be unhelpful, and could actually bring on an attack, perhaps related to the worry or stress induced. It could be 'making it seem more of a problem than it actually is', being 'obsessed' by it or 'wallowing'. As two members explained:

> To get 'strong' and 'above' the problem . . . I needed to forget about it. Meetings drag it all up to the surface.

> Because part of your self-help is not to make too much of a 'thing' about it, so in a way at the meetings you are discussing it a large part of the time. I'm not sure whether that's good or bad.

A few people replied that they were put off attending meetings by coming up against differing viewpoints. One member expressed the criticism that:

> Sometimes the group leaders try to influence you too much that their understanding and morality is the best – not always true.

Some people questioned the whole idea of meeting in a group, of 'meeting strangers with only a virus in common', as one member put it, and felt that it was an artificial or insufficient reason for getting together. A few expressed suspicions or anxieties about people attending groups to look for sexual partners. The possible drawbacks of identification as someone with herpes simplex were cited by 14 per cent as a reason for not going to a group meeting:

I'm not sure I want to accept labelling myself.

It would be an open admission and I still try not to believe it – is this positive thinking?

Public admission would be unhelpful because it would break down my defences.

Ten per cent said simply that they wanted to preserve their anonymity. There was concern about the implications of getting together in this way, several members using the terms 'leper' or 'leper colony'; one member writing that it made one feel 'stigmatised – enhances the feeling that a handicap is present . . . makes one feel abnormal in some way', another suggesting that 'we should not be too inclined to set ourselves apart or [it] will reinforce our ideas that we are somehow different'.

There is clearly a dilemma about meeting other people with a hidden condition in a group. On the one hand, it can allow one to feel 'socially normal' (as one member put it) within the context of the group, because everyone else has the same condition; on the other, getting together with others *because* of the condition can be seen as a statement about one's separateness from the rest of the population – one's abnormality. There is no doubt though, that group meetings can provide something uniquely valuable, expressed by one member as:

The shared experience, strength and hope that can only be found between people who are in the same boat.

NEGOTIATING SEXUAL RELATIONSHIPS

There is contrasting evidence from different investigations of the effect of recurrences of genital HSV symptoms on individuals' sex lives. Among readers of an American journal for people with HSV, a postal survey found that over three-quarters (76 per cent) of the 2,940 respondents felt the way they approached new partners was affected. Most (89 per cent) were concerned about transmitting the infection, and many (69 per cent) feared rejection by a new sexual partner (Catotti, Clarke and Catoe 1993). There was evidence in this investigation that the condition affected respondents' feelings of desirability, as well as their enjoyment and the frequency of sexual intimacy. Asked about the twelve months prior to the survey, 36 per cent of respondents noted a decreased enjoyment of sex and 51 per cent an impact on the frequency of their sexual encounters. These findings echoed those from earlier, smaller surveys. Luby and Klinge (1985), for instance, noted a degree of despair about establishing a 'normal relationship' and that having HSV infection interfered with enjoyment in meeting persons of the opposite sex. They also found 69 per cent of their subjects were fearful of transmitting the condition, 71 per cent had significantly reduced sexual pleasure, 64 per cent inhibited sexual freedom, 47 per cent reduced spontaneity and 47 per cent reduced sexual frequency. Interestingly, they found a bimodal distribution to the answers to the question which asked if having herpes simplex had interfered with sexual enjoyment and intimacy, with 30 per cent saying not at all and another 30 per cent the other end of the scale.

The above findings are clearly from biased samples of the section of the population with symptoms of herpes simplex – those who had identified themselves as 'people with herpes' by joining an organisation for afflicted people or who were attending a physician for medical help with their condition. Among an apparently similar sample in the UK (forty GUM clinic patients and fifty HA members) a different picture was presented by a recent study (Brookes, Haywood and Green 1993) designed to investigate adverse psychological consequences and impaired sexual and interpersonal functioning in people with recurrent genital HSV symptoms. The subjects in this study reported no differences between the frequency of sexual activity currently and prior to the first episode. However, during a current symptomatic episode, sexual activity was reduced (compared to between episodes or prior to the first episode), and during the first six months after diagnosis the frequency of sexual activity was reduced both during and between episodes. There were some subjects who continued sexual activity during episodes. Over the whole sample more subjects (32 per cent) had increased their sexual activity (frequency) since they had first had symptoms of genital HSV infection than had reduced it (22 per cent), half the subjects were in a long-term relationship,

and individuals currently in a sexual relationship reported no reduction in sexual functioning. Furthermore:

> There was no evidence that, for most subjects, having herpes had
> influenced the way in which they saw themselves, their ability to
> relate to others in intimate situations or their feelings of attrac-
> tiveness.
>
> (Brookes, Haywood and Green 1993)

It is in the realm of intimate relationships that this invisible
condition needs to be presented and negotiated. On top of the usual
degree of vulnerability a person may feel on entering a newly intimate relationship, someone with genital symptoms of herpes
simplex has an added vulnerability which may be felt acutely. Even
when recurrences are infrequent, there is a problem associated with
the stigma attached to the condition. Where a person is experiencing frequent recurrences, the physical effects of symptoms may
require some explanation. This leads to anxiety about being
rejected, which, in some people may lead to avoidance of sexual
contact altogether, or to avoidance of telling a partner for as long as
possible and making excuses if they have recurrences, or to having
only casual relationships, and avoiding 'serious' or 'committed' relationships. Another strategy some people have sought in order to
avoid rejection is to look for a sexual partner among the proportion
of the population who identify themselves as 'herpes sufferers'. In
1986, a 'Simplex Dating Service' was set up to put such people in
touch with one another – at the usual dating service cost. An intro-
ductory letter assured that members of the dating service would
have many things in common: the 'need for affection and understanding', having 'gone through periods of physical and . . .
emotional pain . . . rejection and isolation . . . they feel that they
have a right to happiness in life, and . . . they are actively looking
for a solution'. The agency, one of a number of such attempts to get
people together on these grounds, appears to have been unsuccessful
as a business venture and to have closed its books fairly quickly.
Although on the face of it a sensible idea, looked at more closely, it
is less rational. In the first place, the potential partners would need
to know their HSV serotyping in order to be sure that they both
had the same version of the virus: HSV-1 or HSV-2. If one partner
was getting recurrences of HSV-1 (the 'cold sore' version of the
virus) in the genital area and the other had HSV-2, their sexual relationship would expose the first partner to the other version as well

(although antibodies to HSV-1 would provide some protection). If both partners are experiencing frequent episodes of herpetic symptoms at different times, this could result in a far greater interruption of usual sexual activity and possible strain on the relationship, than would be the case with only one partner having such episodes. Potential partners with HSV include not just between a fifth and a third or more of the adult population who have largely asymptomatic HSV-2 infection, but also around 90 per cent of the total adult population who have been infected with HSV-1 (see Chapter 1). Although most of this larger section of the population may not experience symptoms because the virus is dormant, there is the potential for the virus to be reactivated at some point in time when they could pass on the infection via oral sex to anyone who had not previously been in contact with either type of the virus.

The fear of rejection on the part of someone owning up to 'having herpes', is not without some foundation. Most people do not realise the prevalence of HSV infection and that they themselves are more likely than not to have been infected with HSV-1 and to have antibodies as evidence. Their conception of herpes simplex infection on or around the genital area may not be the equivalent of a 'cold sore' in a sensitive place, but a repugnant, incurable, sexually transmitted disease. Their image of the condition and those who have it, may be such that they will not want a relationship with a person who tells them that she or he has intermittent symptoms, let alone take any risk of catching it themselves. Writing about her experiences of hypnotherapy in controlling symptoms, and acceptance in a new-found relationship, an HA member recounts how she had decided six months after diagnosis to tell an old friend about the condition, with the result that:

> He was horrified and disappeared from my life – never to be seen again. I felt like a leper and totally alone. I decided in future I wouldn't tell men that I had a sexual relationship with. It was a terrible pressure and I had to tell lies to try and avoid divulging my secret. I felt more and more alone and incapable of showing affection and contemplated suicide many times.
>
> (*Sphere*, 2: 8)

In accounts of members' personal experiences in the HA newsletter, there were other instances of painful rejections. There were also instances where people reported that they had not suffered rejection and encouraged others to have faith:

One of the most important things I feel I have to share is the positive response I have experienced over the past four years when I have chosen to divulge information about myself re herpes simplex to others, either in a relationship context or otherwise. True, I have never found it easy ... One thing's for sure – the sooner you get a handle on it yourself, the sooner you can deal with the issues of telling other people and feeling in control when you tell them, rather than not being in control and relying on their reactions for making you feel accepted or rejected.

(*Sphere*, 9(3): 12)

The issue of disclosure is one of the most discussed among people getting together because of herpes simplex, and how to tell is the subject of articles and workshops. The advice given tends to cover four main areas: transmission, trust, choosing the right time to tell and giving the other person time to process the information. It is usually not difficult to prevent passing the infection on to someone else since it is not transmissible all the time, but only during recurrences of symptoms (reactivation of the virus), when it is necessary to avoid direct skin-to-skin contact with the affected area. It is more difficult to prevent the transmission of a cold or flu since these infections are airborne. A person who knows they have herpes simplex symptoms will normally be able to recognise signs of a recurrence. The risk of transmission from a person who is aware in this way and acts responsibly is very small (see Chapter 1), and arguably smaller than in the sexually active population at large, among whom there will be a proportion of people who are unaware that they have mild recurrences of HSV symptoms or asymptomatic infection.

In building an ongoing relationship, honesty, trust and mutual caring are clearly important. Not 'telling' may indicate a lack of these qualities in a relationship and this may cause hurt and distrust if the condition is later discovered, particularly if any risks have been taken. Sexual partners have a right to know if they are being exposed to infections which are in any way significant. This means that a person with genital warts (the symptom of human papilloma virus (HPV)) should warn a partner and take the responsibility for having 'safe sex' until the warts are successfully treated, in order not to pass on the infection. A person with recurrences of HSV symptoms in the genital area has a similar responsibility. The risk of transmission can be reduced to a minimum by not having sexual activity during a recurrence. In some cases depending on where the herpetic lesions occur, protection can be gained by the use of a condom and a spermicidal jelly containing nonoxynol-9 which has some antiviral properties. In a world where HIV infection is a potential risk of unprotected sexual intercourse, this strategy would have additional advantages as a routine precaution.

Choosing a suitable time and place for 'telling' is important, as are the words and tone of voice employed in relaying the information. Since herpes simplex is a very common, medically minor and self-limiting condition, using the word 'incurable' is as misleading as using it about chicken pox. Being simply informative is recommended rather than 'lecturing' or 'confessing', particularly about the details of previous sexual relationships. It is recognised that the person's own attitude to themselves and to the condition makes all the difference and is likely to come across in the telling. Thus, it is helpful if the person doing the telling has come to a point of acceptance of the condition in their lives and are not feeling shamed by it, so that they can be as realistic, matter of fact and as calm as possible. There is a need to understand the position of the person being told, to allow them time to take in information, which may be new to them and at variance with what they previously understood, and to deal with any concerns they may have.

Brookes, Haywood and Green (1993) found that the majority (60 per cent) of participants had told their past partners, though 30 per cent said they had not, and most (68 per cent) expected to tell their future partners, though 21 per cent said they were uncertain whether they would tell or not. The study authors commented that:

> more emphasis may need to be given to helping patients to get into a position where they feel able to inform future partners of their infection.
>
> (Brookes, Haywood and Green 1993)

The factors which have a bearing on this situation, are social as much as individual in origin. In order to see this problem in perspective, it needs to be borne in mind that people suffering from 'cold sores' on the lips, may feel upset at the sight or the feel of the symptom, but they do not contemplate suicide, or socially isolate themselves or fear that they will never find a sexual partner who accepts them. Nor do they agonise about how to broach the subject with a potential sexual partner. Yet, this very common expression of

HSV is just as contagious, (and has the potential to be transmitted during sexual activity and result in 'genital' herpes in someone who has not been in contact with the virus before). However, we do not expect a person to warn ' "I had a cold sore last Summer" before s/he kisses you under the mistletoe' (*Sphere*, 3(3): 10)!

Chapter 5

Individual meaning and management

Our knowledge of how individuals experience recurrences of HSV symptoms has come almost entirely from surveys of people attending clinics or belonging to self-help organisations, and volunteers responding to advertisements. These samples have largely been composed of Caucasian young adults who were within the first few years of living with symptoms of HSV infection and had an above average number of recurrences. The majority of research studies have been carried out in the USA. We know very little about the place of herpes simplex in the lives of the majority of people experiencing recurrences who are not seeking medical help or self-help group support, at least not at that point in their lives. As Swanson and Chenitz (1993) have pointed out, there is a gap in knowledge about management of the condition over time. Furthermore, research has focused on psychopathology among people with symptoms in the genital area and not investigated the more common 'lived experience' of herpes simplex, nor included the experiences of those with symptoms on the face, where, because of their visibility, if for no other reason, recurrences may also cause distress. There are some fundamental questions which have hardly been addressed at all, such as how does the average person in the community who is aware of recurrences of HSV, think and feel about this condition, and how much difference does it make if the symptoms appear on one part of the body rather than another? There is considerable evidence that recent diagnosis of HSV infection followed by recurrences of symptoms can significantly impact on the individual's quality of life, although this is not an inevitable accompaniment. After an individual has accommodated to the fact that they have recurrences of HSV symptoms, what kind of impact does herpes simplex have on their quality of life? Is the condition experienced as a significant handicap of any kind? If it is, is the handicap confined to the sphere of sexual relations, and how much does it depend of whether the individual is in a stable relationship?

In order to begin to redress this imbalance in some way, and to encourage a wider view of herpes simplex as a health-related condition, the results of interviews with a small 'community' snowball sample of people will be reviewed as a prelude to discussing the relationship over time between the individual and recurrences of herpes simplex. These individuals had had recurrences of HSV symptoms over a long period ranging from seven to thirty years so that the condition was clearly an ongoing part of their lives. The impact of herpes simplex on their lives was the focus of the inquiry. The interviewees had symptoms on different parts of their bodies: two men and two women had symptoms in the genital area, two women had facial symptoms and one woman had symptoms on her upper arm.

ILLNESS, IMPAIRMENT, DISABILITY OR HANDICAP?

No one interviewed in this community sample thought of herpes simplex as an illness. Asked if they had ever been ill because of HSV, the general answer is summed up in the reply of the man who said:

> Off-colour, but not ill. Sometimes you don't feel one hundred per cent.

However, the first episode was sufficiently severe for three women to remember feeling fairly unwell. One, who had herpes simplex 'all over her face' when she was seventeen, and took two days off work, said that she would have defined herself as ill – 'illness takes over all of me'. Currently the condition causes her 'feelings of discomfort around the face' and 'some emotional lability' once or twice a year. The second, who developed herpes simplex on her upper arm when she started nursing, felt 'ill, sick, general malaise, and tired' with a headache and joint pains bad enough to make her feel she had to rest. Nowadays it causes 'a mild feeling of being unwell, you know there's something wrong but you can't pinpoint it exactly' (until the signs appear). The third woman remembered being at work and feeling suddenly very drained, her work colleagues being concerned because she looked so unwell, and going home feeling awful but unsure what was wrong. A fourth woman, who first developed genital symptoms seven years previously, explained that for the first two years, episodes had been 'flu-like' and caused her to feel like staying in bed, although she had not done so. Thereafter, she had had symptoms infrequently until recently. It can 'make you feel down and irritable' said a male interviewee who had had genital symptoms for twenty-three years. He thought that when he first developed the condition, outbreaks of symptoms:

> seemed to come with 'nerves' and when you've been at your lowest or abused yourself – staying too long at a party.

Likewise, a woman with recurrent herpes simplex symptoms on her face (mouth and nose) was clear that she got the symptoms when she was ill for some reason other than HSV, but the condition itself was not an illness.

A person suffering from a cold might similarly describe their condition as 'not really ill, but not feeling so good today'. There are features of herpes simplex symptom recurrences and colds which help to explain why these conditions are not classed as illnesses. The symptoms in both cases are inconvenient and may be unpleasant but sufferers usually carry on with normal activity. Furthermore, it is known that the symptoms will last a few days and then disappear without any intervention either by the sufferer or a health professional (the condition is self-limiting); and it is also known that the condition is minor and not a threat to the person's current or future health status – it will not worsen and become a more serious condition. Though recurrences of herpes simplex symptoms may be like 'the common cold' in terms of their physical impact, the condition is dissimilar in terms of its potential impact in other dimensions of existence.

A condition may not be thought of as an 'illness' but may nonetheless be located somewhere on the taxonomy of 'impairment', 'disability' or 'handicap' as developed by Wood (1980). Individuals in this community sample were also asked whether they had found having HSV a handicap in personal relationships, and whether they had experienced the condition as an impairment or disability in any other part of life. The overall answer to the first question was ambivalent, but the answer to the second was clearly 'No': in spheres of life other than personal relationships, herpes simplex was not experienced as an impairment or disability. One woman, who had experienced the condition as a handicap in sexual relationships, explained that it had definitely not affected other areas of life and had in fact improved her quality of life in general:

I can't live day to day with a stressful situation. Once I got it, I started to be kinder to myself... There's a lot of things you achieve and you're successful at.

In answer to these questions, the condition was described as 'just an irritation and an embarrassment' by one interviewee, and 'a bloody nuisance' by another, who elaborated on her categorisation by explaining that she had 'always seen it as manageable and it didn't affect any major senses'. A nurse, who called the condition 'a pain in the neck', thought it would be an exaggeration to say that it had been a disability or impairment. She had been required to keep away from neonatal or surgical wards when she had recurrences, although the lesion on her arm would be covered. One interviewee saw HSV as the immediate cause, in the sense of being a trigger, for the condition of postviral fatigue which *had* caused a degree of illness and impairment of function:

I think getting herpes simplex was the last straw on top of all the pressures on me at the time and having had Epstein Barr virus earlier, and it found a hole in my immune system's fence.

The condition had been experienced as a handicap in personal relationships to varying degrees by some of the these interviewees. The two men interviewed who had genital symptoms, had different views of the condition. One said that he found it a handicap in several ways since he had been separated from his wife. For one thing:

You're restricted in what you can do – it affects your sexual performance.

Besides this, he found it difficult to talk about with a prospective partner. He viewed the condition as in the way 'when one wants to go out and enjoy life'. The other male considered that it had not been a handicap and that his ability to form relationships had not suffered. He explained that he had always told his partners, and although the condition 'got in the way of intercourse' it had 'never killed a relationship'. He had 'passed it on' in two cases, but neither of his long-term partners had acquired the condition.

One of the two women interviewed with symptoms in the genital area viewed it as a definite handicap in forming intimate relationships, and as a 'burden' because 'it stays with you all your life' and 'it's always in the back of your mind'. She explained that she tried

not to 'make too big a thing of it' but it was 'not a socially acceptable thing':

> I've come up against a lot of things in life, but this thing, it just –
> I just wish I could put it aside . . . you've got a block there and
> it's stopping you from starting the race.

She believed in telling her partners and thought that a man would
not necessarily be deterred by it, if only because he might not be
fully aware of the impact it could have on his life. However, she had
felt restricted by the responsibility she felt. She added that she
thought of HSV as:

> an amber light which stopped you from getting anything worse.

This image of the indicator which is neither a complete halt to
proceeding, nor a green light, but a warning, probably reflects an
aspect of many individuals' attitude to having acquired HSV in the
genital area. The other woman with symptoms on the lower part of
her body area did not consider the condition any kind of handicap
to forming sexual relationships. However, her recurrences had been
infrequent, and usually on the back of the thigh where they could
be covered with a plaster to prevent contact, or at the base of the
spine. She said:

> Why worry about herpes simplex when there are far more serious
> viral infections around which can kill you?

Symptoms of herpes simplex occurring on the face can also be
experienced as something of a handicap or limitation – socially and
sexually. When one interviewee first got symptoms, she was a self-
conscious adolescent:

> The way I used to get them was hideous. I'm less likely to hide
> away now . . . I no longer look like I've just come out of a leper
> colony.

Although she is 'not too thrilled about the way it looks on my
mouth', an outbreak of herpetic symptoms nowadays would not
stop her going out. Another interviewee with intermittent facial
symptoms would limit her sexual activity, precluding oral sex
during an outbreak.

The interviewee with herpes simplex recurrences on her upper
arm consoled herself that it was not on her face, but still felt there
was 'a certain stigma attached to it', and thought that it looked 'so

horrible', but felt covering it was like 'another label'. She tried to wear clothes that covered the area because, even after having it for thirty years, she did not like people commenting on it. Her husband had not been worried about it, nor any of her friends, but she felt it had 'the potential to be a problem in a relationship'.

CHANGING VIEWS AND MEANING FOR THE INDIVIDUAL

A person's view of HSV is likely to change over the time elapsed since the first symptoms were experienced (Chapter 3), and according to their changed circumstances.

> When I first got it, I thought it was the end of the world . . . then it just became a nuisance . . . I knew what it was and I just had to live with it.
>   (Male interviewee with genital symptoms for twenty-three years)

For the other man interviewed, it had only become a problem when his marriage had broken up two years previously. During the ten years prior to that, he had only had symptoms once or twice a year. The subsequent stress and changes in his life appeared to be associated with more frequent recurrences and he was now finding this a restriction as a single man. 'Initially it was shock, horror and I thought I was going to die' explained a female interviewee who felt that she had subsequently, but only for a time, come to terms with having genital symptoms of the condition – 'Now I've lost the plot a bit'. Living with a fellow sufferer whom she met in a support group had allowed a respite from the concerns she felt about forming sexual relationships. However, she later felt 'the only thing we had in common was herpes' and that she was allowing the condition to determine her choices in life: 'I was making decisions because of it'. She saw suppressive treatment as allowing her greater freedom of choice, and, in terms of her metaphor of life as 'playing the game', perhaps as providing a more even playing field:

> You play the game . . . if you're not playing at all, you're doing nothing about negotiating your place.

Viewing the condition as a considerable 'burden', she had changed her view of what else she felt she could cope with in life:

> I can't take on a man who's on drugs or drink or has problems.

Now I'm saying I can't help people to make changes . . . If there's no good situation around, I won't take on a bad situation.

The attitude of the other female with symptoms on the lower half of her body to the virus had twice changed. The first time was when she made the connection between her primary episode and the development of post-viral fatigue-like illness. She thereafter considered that herpes simplex had been her nemesis, rather than an occasional nuisance with no significant consequences. The second time was when she had thought the recurrences had stopped, but then had to face the fact that they had simply moved their site:

I didn't get symptoms in the usual places any more and I was triumphant and thought 'Great, I've beaten it at last'. And then I realised it hadn't disappeared at all and there it was, every now and then, one or two little vesicles hiding away at the bottom of my spine. I thought 'You little beast'!

The female interviewee who first developed symptoms on her arm in her second year as a student nurse had been 'quite upset about it'. Her father had had difficulty accepting that the infection was not curable and had wanted to sue the hospital. She herself had eventually come to an acceptance:

You can't do anything about it, you might as well put up with it.

Her concerns about the condition had centred on 'giving it to somebody else' or 'catching something on top of it'. (As the area of vesicles was sometimes large and could get 'weepy', like an ulcer, there was always the possibility of the lesion being infected). As a mother she had worried about transmitting the condition to her children.

Of the two female interviewees who had had facial symptoms since adolescence, one came from a family where the condition was an accepted part of life, as the mother 'gets them really badly . . . right across her face', and all of her four children also have obvious symptoms. This interviewee became concerned, however, when she started getting symptoms in her nose because it was painful and she worried that the symptoms might one day progress further and she would get meningitis. (She would have antibodies to HSV-1, and unless she developed severe immunosuppression, recurrences would only occur facially). The other interviewee had taken a range of preventive measures which she believed to be helpful over the years, but accepted that once a recurrence had occurred:

I know whatever I do they'll last a week . . . I've learnt to coexist with it.

One of the most difficult aspects of this coexistence, was the tendency for symptoms to occur at the time when 'something important was coming up', and this caused her considerable angst because she knew 'this grand event would be accompanied by cold sores'. She summed up her feelings about recurrences which she viewed as a sign that she was 'out of balance':

I feel annoyed and inconvenienced and crabby . . . resentment and irritation.

Having lived with symptoms of HSV for twenty-six years, however, she had attributed a meaningful role in her life to the condition:

It's my lot . . . I guess it's teaching me something. It's teaching me humility. It's a spiritual lesson – that I can't be less than perfect.

From these interviews with people who were aware that they had had the condition over many years, we can see that herpes simplex was largely experienced as a minor condition producing intermittent, inconvenient symptoms, and that it was interwoven with the intimate fabric of people's lives, an unwelcome accompaniment to big events, an amber light in sexual relations, something to be covered up, a barometer of one's emotional and physical state and an intermittent reminder of one's imperfection. People attach their own meanings to this condition which has acquired significant social meaning (Chapter 1). They may or may not take on the socially stigmatised meaning at some stage, but their experience of the condition will be affected by their current circumstances, so that the meaning has different layers reflecting different factors (individual, societal, contextual) that make up the significance of the condition at that point in the individual's life.

It is frequently the case that HSV is one problematic factor in the middle of interrelated changes in sexual partnerships. One account of a personal experience in the Herpes Association's newsletter *Sphere* (8(4): 12) explained how the author discovered her HSV infection and her fiancé's unfaithfulness around the same time. The two interlinked traumas were both implicated in her feelings of being 'betrayed, grief-stricken and angry . . . utterly torn apart and destroyed' each making the other more painful and difficult to bear.

She had monthly recurrences of HSV genital symptoms which left her 'depressed and debilitated' so that she:

> reached such an all-time low of self-pity and shame that I was even considering if it was worth going on . . . When you're sore, feeling shameful, dirty and suffering from frequent recurrences it is difficult to get HSV into some kind of perspective.

It was at this time, a turning point in her relationship with HSV, that she made contact with the HA which was 'a real lifeline' and then went on a three-month course of suppressive therapy prescribed by her GP. This woman's personal circumstances at the time clearly affected her experience of herpes simplex infection.

A presenter at the HA's press conference on 16 June 1993, Marian Benson, described how she experienced a change in the meaning to her of her condition from the mid-1970s, when she first experienced genital symptoms, to the mid-1980s when her view of it had become much more negative as a result of being influenced by the media presentation. When the infection was diagnosed she was told simply that she had 'herpes simplex, the name for the virus that causes cold sores', that it would go away by itself and she should not have sex while it was present. She had the occasional sore every ten months or so, but was not particularly concerned about or troubled by them. In the early 1980s, however, she came across an article in *Time* magazine which presented herpes simplex recurrences, which she had thought of as 'merely cold sores on my genitals' as 'a fearsome and loathsome disease':

> A disease! 'Any impairment of normal physiological function caused by infection' . . . My cold sores impaired me a good deal less than my 'skiing knee' as far as normal physiological functioning went. All sorts of other words attached themselves to my innocent cold sores: 'curse of the promiscuous' . . . 'incurable' . . . 'sufferers' . . . 'epidemic'.
>
> (Marian Benson, Herpes Association press briefing, 16 June 1993)

She found that 'growing fear and horror [was] taking over my thoughts' and worried that no one who knew that she had recurrences of HSV symptoms would ever want a sexual relationship with her. She had many recurrences at this time. Although the tube of anaesthetic gel given her in the clinic where she had been diagnosed meant that she did not 'hurt physically':

psychologically, I was hurting like hell . . . For a period of about a year, I wondered if a life with no prospect of a sexual relationship was actually worth living . . . Luckily my hectic job was also very interesting and kept me going.

(ibid.)

Through subsequent contact with the HA, information and group meetings:

gradually herpes simplex was put back into perspective. And as it fell into perspective, the episodes died away.

(ibid.)

In this case, the different social contexts in which Marian experienced herpes simplex can be seen to have influenced both how she thought about the condition and how it affected her.

In effect, people with recurrent HSV symptoms have a relationship with this intermittent visitor to their bodily surface and consciousness. The individual's response to such visitations can vary from paying very little, if any, attention, to constant preoccupation with the threat and meaning attributed to them. The frequency and severity of symptoms will have a significant, but not determining, influence on this response. A person with mild and infrequent recurrences may have a strong and continuing reaction to the threat of them and the meaning of 'living with HSV' in his or her life. This, in turn, will be influenced by individual and social factors and the immediate context in which they are experienced. In this respect, the experience of recurrences of HSV symptoms as a chronic condition is like very many other bodily conditions related to a person's health in that it is not straightforwardly correlated with the biomedical symptoms or signs. To account for and more completely understand the experience of symptoms, it is therefore insufficient to pay attention only to the physical features. As discussed above, a person's view of the condition, and thus response, may change as the circumstances in which they are experienced, change.

THE INDIVIDUAL RESPONSE TO RECURRENCES

In a bid to have some control over symptom recurrences and the impact of the condition on his or her life, an individual may use various means to influence the processes which lead to their occurrence. The extent to which the interviewees in this community sample had sought and used medical intervention, or themselves tried to prevent recurrences, varied between one individual and another, and from one time in their life to another. The female interviewee with recurrences on her arm had sought medical help and been given four or five successive smallpox vaccinations in an attempt to boost her immune system's response to HSV in 1975. She thought this treatment had not helped. She had also tried Zovirax cream when it became available, but had found it was not effective for her. She now simply uses Betadine to prevent infection of the lesion. Of the two females who had facial symptoms, one had not sought medical help but went to considerable trouble to try to prevent outbreaks of symptoms, keeping the sun off her face by wearing a hat, and using No. 15 sunblock on her nose and lips, and consciously managing stress in her life by increased resting and meditation. She had also taken L-lysine tablets 'prophylactically'. The other interviewee with facial symptoms had mentioned the condition to her GP who offered to prescribe her acyclovir if the recurrences became more of a problem. She expressed reluctance about taking suppressive medication. (The normal frequency of her recurrences was three times a year or less, but in the last few months recurrences had been more frequent and accompanied upper respiratory tract viral infections). Adjusting her lifestyle to try to avoid recurrences was not her approach:

> If I go to the beach, it triggers it, but I don't let that stop me . . . I don't really do anything to prevent them. I always forget that I get them.

Of the two male interviewees with genital symptoms, one had not sought medical help since his initial diagnosis. He related recent outbreaks of symptoms to stress, but said he had no time to try stress reduction techniques. He thought it important that he took a lot of vitamins and had always kept to a balanced diet. The other male with genital symptoms had tried a whole range of medical treatments in the 1970s and '80s. He had regularly used Idoxuridine solution. At a time when he had been getting very regular recurrences, he was given superficial X-ray therapy (SXRT) to the genital area and was required to take himself to the clinic in a central London hospital as soon as he felt the beginning of a recurrence. He also took things into his own hands:

> With me nothing seemed to work . . . I used to get a hot needle and burst the blisters thinking I was easing it.

When Zovirax was first available, he used the ointment and took tablets as suppressive treatment for six months. Currently he takes Zovirax tablets during recurrences.

One of the female interviewees with genital symptoms had recently decided to go on suppressive treatment in order to feel 'freer', in her terms, to seek a sexual partnership. The other female with symptoms in the lower half of her body had on occasions used Zovirax cream, but had come to the conclusion that it made no difference to the length of time an outbreak took to heal. The early pattern of her recurrences appeared predetermined since they came twice a year at the same point in the calendar each time. Then the pattern of recurrences changed, and they were milder and associated with tiredness or illness. She regularly took vitamin C and zinc supplements, as much for her 'general' health as to help prevent recurrences, and tried to ensure that she had enough sleep. She had sometimes experienced prodromal pain going down her leg or elsewhere on her torso and, before there was any sign of any actual outbreak on the skin, she would try 'mind over matter – telling it very firmly to "get lost" '.

When they were asked if there were ways they could help themselves, Herpes Association (HA) group members interviewed in 1987 (see Chapter 3) also revealed very different views and approaches. A distinction was made between physical and emotional help, one member saying that:

> dealing with it physically [there's] nothing to be done; dealing with it emotionally it's a problem of relationships.

A fundamental difference of approach between one implying that attempted control of recurrences was a mistake and one which held that it was quite possible to intervene helpfully was also evident:

> Not really something you can do anything about. It's a matter of just relaxing and letting things be – letting nature take its course. The more I worried about it, the more I was getting it.

> As a long-term sufferer I know what triggers an attack, and what to do to widen the gaps between attacks. I feel I have considerable control.

Most of the interviewees' answers were in line with this latter approach and implied that there were things one could do to minimise attacks. The suggested ways of helping oneself focused on various ways of reducing stress (going to bed, relaxing, calming down, Alexander technique and Tai Chi), boosting the immune system ('a whole person approach must assist your overall health and herpes'), and a variety of complementary therapies (deep-cleansing diet, colonics, homeopathy, herbalism). Care and manipulation of the body was not the only way of controlling the physical expression of HSV – manipulation of the mind in the form of hypnotherapy was also mentioned by a member who said that it had resulted in a better attitude to his health:

> I've become healthier because of having herpes. I try to control the way I think about it.

The evidence from the survey of HA members presented in Chapter 3 (Posner 1990), suggested that people have idiosyncratic strategies for managing their recurrences, which tend to be constructed from elements which are common to many, but which are combined in an individual way. Many of the elements of strategies to prevent recurrences such as stress reduction, sufficient rest, a balanced diet, avoidance of excess in physical terms, and a positive attitude to life, are common to health-promoting/maintaining strategies in general. Thus, acknowledgement of a problem of HSV symptom recurrences may result in the individual becoming more health conscious, more aware of their own physical limitations and concerned to look after their bodily selves, in order not to be inconvenienced by an outbreak of HSV symptoms.

> At times I'm pleased to have had the herpes experience. Perhaps I'm glamorising this, conveniently forgetting some of the anxieties I suffered at the time and instead concentrating on the positive learning experience. I became more aware of my own stress patterns, more responsible for my own health.
>
> (*Sphere*, 8(4): 11)

RESEARCH STUDIES OF THE RELATIONSHIP BETWEEN PSYCHOSOCIAL FACTORS AND RECURRENCES

There have been many attempts to sort out the complex interrelationships between psychosocial factors, particularly stress and social support, psychometric variables and the experience of HSV symptom recurrences. In general, these investigations have demonstrated associations and suggested mediating variables without directly addressing causality. From their review of this literature, Longo and Koehn (1993) concluded:

Psychosocial factors such as stress (life events and hassles), emotional distress (anxiety, depression, anger and obsessionality), personality (Type A and self-esteem), attributions (coping and internality), and social support are significantly associated with genital herpes recurrence rates or HSV episode severity and duration. Several mediating factors (internality, disease duration, social support, and illness vulnerability) have also been shown to be important in the prediction of herpes outbreaks and the nature of the HSV episode.

A number of these investigations have been correlational studies using retrospective designs. Goldmeier and Johnson (1982) investigated fifty-eight patients with primary genital herpes and found that patients with high scores for psychiatric symptoms (anxiety, depression, and obsessional thinking using the General Health Questionnaire (GHQ)) experienced significantly more recurrences of HSV symptoms over a thirty-week period than individuals with low psychiatric symptom scores. Subsequent studies by these authors also found the same positive association between recurrences and psychiatric symptoms. Stout and Bloom (1986) demonstrated that among the thirty-four women in their study, those with a higher number of recurrences had higher mean values on nine of the ten subscales of the Minnesota Multiphasic Personality Inventory, and were more depressed, anxious, tense, hostile, impulsive, preoccupied with health concerns and socially alienated than those with a lower number of recurrences. Manne and Sandler (1984) also found positive correlations between psychosocial factors and the annual number of HSV symptom recurrences, but the nature of the association varied with the length of time the subject had had the condition: where this was less than a year, stress was positively correlated with recurrences; where this was longer than a year, depression and poor self-esteem were positively correlated with the number of yearly recurrences. Lacroix and Offutt (1988) found no difference in the HSV genital symptom recurrence rates between subjects classed as 'Type A' and 'Type B' personality, though those with 'Type A' personality reported more severe symptoms.

Other retrospective studies using multiple regression analysis have demonstrated the mediating effects of duration of the condi-

tion, locus of control, social support, and 'coping' on the relationships between recurrences of HSV symptoms and stress and/or
emotional distress. Watson (1983) found that recent life stress (as
measured by the Life Experiences Scale) and recurrences of HSV
symptoms were positively correlated and that internal locus of
control and social support functioned as a mediating variable, so
that study participants who were high on internality and/or social
support were less likely to have an increased number of recurrences
regardless of their level of stressful life events. In the study by
VanderPlate, Aral and Magder (1988), positive relationships were
also found between recent life stress and recurrences of HSV symptoms, but this relationship was mediated by social support and the
duration of HSV infection, so that it only applied where the person
had had the condition for less than four years or when 'herpes-
specific' social support was low. A relationship was not found
between recent life stress (as measured by the Life Experiences
Scale) and frequency of recurrences or emotional dysfunction (as
measured by the Symptom Checklist-90) by Silver et al. (1986).
However, their regression analysis indicated that higher frequencies
of recurrence, and greater discomfort related to symptoms, were
associated with an external locus of control orientation, a tendency
to use emotion-focused wishful thinking, and to avoid using cognitive strategies (such as minimisation of threat) as a way of coping
with stress associated with herpes simplex. High levels of emotional
dysfunction were found and these were associated with the
frequency, pain and 'bother' of symptom recurrences. Levenson et
al. (1987) found that psychological factors (depression, anxiety,
somatisation, interpersonal sensitivity and life change) were more
predictive of pain and itching related to symptom episodes than
were somatic indices such as duration of the episode and rate of
annual HSV recurrences. The findings of the study by Longo and
Clum (1989) were in line with many of the above-mentioned associations. These authors reported that relationships between symptom
episode duration and severity was predicted by severity of
emotional distress, and that an internal health locus of control was
negatively associated with episode severity. They also found that
annual rates of genital HSV symptoms were 'positively associated
with and predicted by stress and emotional distress', and demonstrated that duration of the condition and internal locus of control
had a mediating effect (so that stress had the greatest effect in those
who had had the condition for a shorter time).

Two prospective studies failed to demonstrate a *direct* relationship between stress and recurrences of HSV symptoms. Rand et al. (1990) followed sixty-four individuals with genital HSV symptoms from one to three months evaluating stress factors in their daily life and the occurrence of symptoms. They found no significant correlations between normal daily stress (psychological/emotional, physical health, educational/vocational, financial and interpersonal relationships) and recurrences of HSV symptoms. However, the study did not address mediating effects, and may have included subjects for whom stress was not a trigger for symptom recurrences. A study by Kemeny et al. (1989) conducted for six months on forty-six individuals with recurrent genital symptoms of herpes simplex, investigated stress, mood, social support and immunocompetence in relation to symptom recurrences. This study found significant correlations between high stress and low immunocompetence and between high negative mood (anxiety, depression and hostility) and low immunocompetence. Stress was not a predictor of recurrences; however, there was a highly significant positive correlation between depression and HSV recurrences for the most depressed subjects in the study. These investigators suggested that subjects with higher trait depression may be more vulnerable to stress-induced HSV symptom recurrences, whether the stress is physical or psychological, due to lower immunocompetence. In their causal model, Hoon et al. (1991) used the related concept of 'illness vulnerability' (defined by the occurrence of non-herpes illness during the study), and suggested that this was linked directly to symptom recurrences and that stress and social support indirectly influenced symptom recurrences via illness vulnerability.

Carney and colleagues (Carney et al. 1993, 1994) questioned the hypothesis that stress or an individual's emotional state caused recurrences, and argued that it was the frequency of the physical manifestations of the condition that made the difference to psychological response. Their study, looking at the effect on psychiatric morbidity of suppressive treatment for patients with frequently recurring genital symptoms (Carney et al. 1993), found that the percentage of GHQ cases fell from 63 per cent initially to 26 per cent three months after the commencement of treatment. Illness concern and hospital anxiety measured on the Hospital Anxiety and Depression Questionnaire was also reduced significantly. These findings may relate to psychological responses to apparent control of the condition, as much as to the absence of physical symptoms, and do not preclude the influence of psychosocial factors on symptom recurrence in the absence of suppressive treatment.

In a study investigating coping responses, Keller, Jadack and Mims (1991) found that the number of recurrences per year was not related to perceived disease-related stressors. Study participants with very low recurrence rates reported as many disease-related stressors as those with high recurrence rates. Moreover, none of the sixty participants in this study reported that symptoms were the most upsetting disease-related stressor. In a further analysis of the data collected in this study (Jadack, Keller and Hyde 1990), it was demonstrated that disease activity influenced the perceived impact of the condition, so that Keller, Jadack and Mims (1991) concluded that 'the role of disease activity in overall adjustment is much more complex than previous literature would suggest'. Indeed, while the interconnection between the biopsychosocial factors related to HSV symptom recurrences has been amply demonstrated, the matrix is complicated with mediating variables such as social support and duration of the condition, influencing the impact of stress or depression. Even in the frequently assumed association between stress or emotional distress and more frequent recurrences of HSV symptoms, the directionality of any causal connection which may exist in some, but not all, individuals is unclear.

THE UPWARD HERPES SIMPLEX ILLNESS TRAJECTORY

When Strauss (1975) used the concept of 'trajectory' in relation to chronic diseases, he suggested that most are moving downward (towards increased illness or disability), but that they varied in their predictability and the shape of their downward course. The recurrence of symptoms of HSV infection is very uncertain in general, although in a particular individual it can become more predictable over time. The condition is different from many other chronic conditions, however, in that trajectories move upwards – people tend to suffer its symptoms less and less often and the symptoms tend to become less acute. The upward-moving trajectory may plateau at a certain point, after which the individual's experience of symptoms remains the same. Sometimes, the trajectory may dip downwards for a time, and people can be troubled by symptoms again after a long period in which they were absent. The overall trend (except in people whose immune systems are seriously compromised) is towards improvement.

Alongside the physical signs of improvement, is the individual's process of adaptation which involves coming to terms with the idea of HSV infection and its implications. This psychosocial process is very much influenced by the individual's view of the condition, as illustrated above (and in Chapter 3), and by the individual's circumstances as discussed above (and in Chapter 4), and it may proceed at a faster or slower pace than the biophysical adaptation. The meaning of the condition at a particular point in the life of an individual with recurrences, and any management strategies adopted, will both reflect and, in turn, have an effect on these processes.

Chapter 6

Fighting stigma

Self-help organisations bring people together either literally, in groups of people who meet each other, usually on a regular basis, or in some other form of fellowship. The organisation is then in a position through its main office or central point, its key officer or officers, to represent its members by acting and speaking on their behalf. This representational and advocacy role of self-help organisations takes different forms according to the nature of the condition involved and the development of the organisation. With a group organised around a condition which carries a stigma in the wider society, activity will be focused on *re-presenting* the condition to the members of the group in a less negative way, and on trying to change the societal image of the condition and its bearers. The UK Herpes Association (HA) has both represented the interests of those who are troubled in body or mind by the symptoms, and tried to re-present the nature of the problem to the population at large and to the members of the association in order to counteract the stigma associated with the genital form of the condition. The dissemination of information has been crucial to this activity.

THE FORMATION OF THE HERPES ASSOCIATION

The Herpes Association in London began in a way typical of self-help groups with a few people with the condition getting together. The process started with an advertisement asking to meet others with HSV placed in *Spare Rib* by Sue Blanks in early 1980. There were five replies, one from another woman living in London. They met each other and for the first time talked with another person suffering with herpes simplex symptoms and found great solidarity and reassurance. They wrote about their experiences in an article for

Spare Rib in late 1980. The response to this article resulted in the organisation of the first self-help group meeting for women only in London in 1981. The group continued to meet, Sue Blanks and Carole Woddis contributed to media coverage of herpes simplex at this time, and another member of the original group started a mixed sex group after placing an advertisement in the personal columns of *Time Out*. It became clear from the response to this activity, that something more than informal support groups was needed. The Herpes Association was set up and launched at a conference in November 1982. Nine months later there were eight local groups, 3,000 people had been helped with replies to their letters, and the group contact for the association (which was still housed with *Spare Rib* but applying for charitable status), could write:

> The medical profession is beginning to recognise us as an established, responsible and knowledgeable organisation. Invitations have come to speak at Special Clinics . . . as well as to medical students and other groups.

The HA became a Registered Charity in 1985 and received its first funding grant. The organisation was run by a management committee drawn from the membership and an executive officer was appointed who remained in that post for a decade. The association received grants from the Department of Health as well as the London Boroughs Grants Committee.

EXPERIENTIAL INFORMATION AS A RESOURCE

Having one continuing key officer of the association for over a decade meant that very considerable experience and knowledge of the condition was acquired through his contacts with thousands of people. The association's officer functioned as an information broker, exchanging medically accepted knowledge acquired from medical journals, books and contacts, with the observations and experiences of people living with the condition. This interactive process, he suggested, had been a 'gradual, slow sifting process' which had resulted in himself and the HA office becoming a 'central pool of information'. This knowledge base was different from medical expertise, but was nonetheless a form of expertise of the sort acquired by health-related self-help organisations from the myriad of personal experiences of members and people contacting the organisation with the condition.

We have handled more than 60,000 enquiries over the years, and have a unique picture of what actually happens.

(Mike Wolfe, HA, quoted in *Sunday Times*, 20 June 1993)

In an interview with Mike Wolfe, the executive officer of the Herpes Association, in September 1993, he described how, when he came into the job, he began finding discrepancies between different authorities and between the reported 'facts' on HSV and what he was hearing from people with symptoms of the condition.

I suppose in very simple terms, it was a matter of observing what actually happened in relation to what we were told was happening, or the concerns which we were told we should be observing – mainly by the lay press – and they just didn't fit, didn't quite add up.

(Mike Wolfe, personal communication)

This, in effect, led to a 'deconstruction' of the condition of herpes simplex as presented in the media, particularly the lay press of the early 1980s. Ideas about transference, auto-inoculation, pregnancy and childbirth, links with cervical cancer, the nature of the 'epidemic' and the media's preoccupation with genitalia were all critically examined.

It was a matter of all this information filtering and gradually from that, you build up a picture of what is really going on in the physiological sense as opposed to what we're told happens, and then separating very clearly the physiological and psychological aspects, although they're clearly interrelated in terms of recurrences.

(Mike Wolfe, personal communication)

The re-presentation of herpes simplex based on this accumulated evidence took place in a number of ways over a period of some years – initially by giving information to journalists writing articles for the popular press, or writing to try to correct the misinformation given in such articles; then by the publication of a comprehensive booklet (the second issued by the association); and finally in a press conference. Throughout this time, the association's newsletter contained information for members on a range of topics, and, particularly in the 1990s, some authoritative and comprehensive articles summarising accumulated knowledge about an aspect of living with HSV.

One such article 'Pregnancy and Childbirth – The Unkindest Cut . . . ' (*Sphere*, 8: 1) discussed the evidence and issues relating to HSV, pregnancy and childbirth. The executive officer described the process of putting this article together, using British Paediatric Surveillance Unit data, 'posing questions rather than presenting opinions' – his aim being responsibly to present information for parents to make choices:

> So all in all, the whole thing . . . took probably somewhere in the region of two and a half years of painstakingly asking questions, of double-checking and talking to all . . . sorts of people, and finally getting to the point where I felt safe and secure in the information I put down – not to be in any way detrimental to the mother or baby.

The article is an example of the combining of epidemiological, medical and experiential information gathered by the association. It was introduced with 'A midwife's observations' mostly covering the unwanted consequences of Caesarean sections, but also commenting:

> The facts are quite clearly stated that as long as at the time of delivery the woman is not experiencing a primary infection she can proceed with a normal delivery as long as her pregnancy is full term . . . by this time the baby will have built up its own immunity to the virus.
>
> (*Sphere*, 8(1): 1)

In 1993, the association was still hearing from pregnant women who were told or had read that they would require a Caesarean delivery of their baby simply because they had a history of genital HSV symptoms. The article went on to acknowledge that medical attitudes and practices were changing and to suggest that prospective mothers could challenge any insistence on their having a Caesarean delivery on those grounds alone. It argued that women should be informed of the known risks of Caesarean sections and allowed to weigh them up against the hypothetical risks of HSV transmission during birth. The reasons for such a challenge were that Caesarean operations themselves carry a risk for the mother, and that the evidence available, indicates that full-term babies born to mothers with a history of HSV symptoms are at very low risk of infection (see 'The Biomedical Context' section in Chapter 1) so that the likelihood would be that the operation would be unnecessary. The article quoted the 1991 Annual Report of the British Paediatric Surveillance Unit which recorded thirteen neonatal infections with HSV out of approximately three-quarters of a million births, with four neonatal deaths due to HSV; over 70 per cent of the mothers of infected babies have no history of symptoms of HSV infection; HSV types 1 and 2 are equally responsible for neonatal infection and death. The article suggested that if the baby is vulnerable to primary infection because it has no antibody protection, it is equally at risk from a relative's kiss or skin contact with a nurse shedding the virus. The association had accumulated evidence of this happening:

> During the past 10 years, myself, colleagues and helpliners have listened to the experiences of many thousands of women. To date not one has reported that they have infected their baby. In contrast to this, I have talked with seven women whose babies were infected and died. None of these seven had a history of HSV or evidence of antibody presence.
>
> (*Sphere*, 8(1): 5)

The article concluded that there was 'what one could almost describe as a conspiracy of silence on this issue. Thus allowing the doom merchants to have centre stage. . . . Some clear and official direction on this matter [was] long overdue'. In its absence there were many unnecessary Caesareans and the issue was 'far more contentious . . . than it need be'.

The association's second comprehensive booklet *Herpes Simplex. A Guide* issued in 1993, also drew on the accumulation of evidence from the association's members and contacts. Its writing required a 'very slow process (involving) double checking, doubts, asking and re-asking'. The executive officer felt he 'had to be more careful to be accurate than a doctor, because he would stand up to be knocked down more easily'. In talking about HSV, he was often asked if he was medically qualified. The suggestion that the common experience of this widespread infection could only be spoken about with authority by a medically qualified person is ironical in the case of a condition which is so widely experienced in the population, but typical of the undervaluation of experiential, as opposed to biomedical information relating to chronic conditions. On the back cover of the booklet was the acknowledgement, 'The information in this booklet is based on the actual experiences of tens of thousands of individuals'.

THE IDEOLOGICAL BATTLE

The dissemination of information about the condition of herpes simplex has tended to be very much intertwined with the ideological position of the informant. It was the genital version of HSV which acquired a popular significance and became embedded in the cultural reworking of morals and attitudes towards sexual freedom. Analytically, it is possible to find ideological components in the popular presentations of many medical conditions, in the sense of different stances towards a condition with different implications for action. Writing about living with multiple sclerosis (MS), Robinson pointed to the difference between the stance of the MS Society and that of ARMS (Action for Research into Multiple Sclerosis), an organisation whose position was more representative of those who 'feel they want more active involvement in the management of their disease through direct control of the direction and implementation of medical policy and practice' (Robinson 1988: 119). The ideological component of presentations of HSV in the media has been very considerable and has covered the very nature of herpes simplex, not just prescriptions for action. The condition has been fought over in ideological terms, particularly in relation to its (medical and social) significance, with implications for how those who clearly have the condition are viewed, how risks of transmission should be treated, and the need or otherwise of medical intervention.

By the early 1990s, the HA was being regularly consulted by journalists when they wrote articles about herpes simplex. The association was able to have some influence on the information in the lay press and to begin to get across the message that the presentation of herpes simplex in the media had been seriously distorted and had adversely affected people's experience of the condition. An article by Frances Hubbard in the *Daily Express* (17 October 1990), headlined 'Whatever happened to the herpes plague?', suggested:

> The truth is that herpes has existed for at least 2000 years without posing any serious threat to humanity . . . Most (people) live happily with it without suffering a single symptom.

It later quoted a representative (Mike Wolfe) of the HA saying that ignorance causes pointless anguish, the psychological effects can be worse than the physical ones, and that 'the epidemic of media distortion about herpes was bigger than the real thing'. The

Guardian Women's Section also carried an article (by Memuna Forna, 30 May 1991) suggesting that the 'herpes hype . . . reporting herpes as a sexual scourge visited on the promiscuous left a legacy of misunderstanding which . . . has done more to cause anguish to sufferers than their minor skin disorder'. The article quoted another representative of the HA saying:

> People . . . with genital herpes were subjected to a barrage of sensationalism in the early eighties which added a major psychological dimension to their mainly minor physical problems . . . the stigma attached to genital herpes is all the more ridiculous when you consider it is as old as man himself and survey after survey has shown up to 90 per cent of adults carry the virus. But because the majority of these carriers have facial infections or are symptom-free, it is the unlucky minority who shoulder the stigma.

An *Esquire* article (by Sarah Stacey, September 1993) made the point directly with the headline 'Herpes owes its bad name to the media – not to its symptoms'. This was followed by the suggestion from yet another representative of the HA that:

> We have all been conditioned over the last couple of decades to overreact . . . Herpes is really a minor condition which was completely hyped up by the media during the Seventies and Eighties.

The article went on to quote a doctor from a GUM unit saying:

> The biggest problem is psychological. The symptoms are sometimes very distressing, but they can be controlled and complications are rare.

As far as GPs were concerned, herpes simplex had come from being a condition that many doctors took little notice of because it was common, minor and self-limiting, to one which was presented as the ruination of a person's life, the cause of suicidal feelings and great distress and thus requiring intervention – symptom alleviation, symptom suppression, counselling or at least reassurance. This is reflected in Wellcome advertisements which portrayed their product Zovirax as rescuing people with recurrent genital symptoms of HSV from their plight. For instance, adverts in the medical press heralding the greater freedom of doctors in Australia to prescribe Zovirax tablets from the beginning of December 1993 showed a photograph of a woman dancing in the air, with the words 'doctor frees unfairly imprisoned woman' in large letters over the picture. It continued:

For thousands of Australians, recurrent genital herpes can be a cruel sentence of pain and distress. The only effective way to free these patients and give back control of their lives is with Zovirax (acyclovir) . . . As a doctor, you can offer this freedom.

In another advertisement announcing these more relaxed prescribing regulations for Zovirax, the caption read:

Recurrent genital herpes can cause profound psychological, emotional and sexual dysfunction. From the patient's point of view it is incurable and stigmatising.

And prominence was given to a table of 'significant life areas affected by genital herpes recurrences' which included self-concept, emotional life, interpersonal relations, sexual functioning and work or school adapted from a paper by Drob, Loemer and Lifshutz (1985). Yet another advert in the medical press around this time showed men and women chained to the poles of a merry-go-round under the heading 'How much longer will they be trapped by the recurrences of genital herpes?' The advertisement read:

For genital herpes patients who experience frequent recurrences, Zovirax offers freedom from the cycle of pain and discomfort but more importantly, from the fear and apprehension that often traps them.

While the medical profession was being persuaded that people suffering recurrent genital HSV symptoms were deserving of sympathy and medical help, the HA in the UK was effectively countering the earlier stigmatised media presentation of 'genital' herpes, getting across the message that the condition was not medically serious and down-playing the likely effect on a person's life. At the same time, a new 'health education campaign' was telling people that 'cold sores' were highly contagious and just as dangerous as the genital version of herpes simplex – but treatment was available. An article in the *Evening Standard* (by Lois Rogers, 30 October 1991) announced the Cold Sore Education Campaign in language reminiscent of the articles on genital symptoms of herpes simplex in the early 1980s:

Alarm over Aids has masked a massive explosion in cases of the cold sore virus herpes which can cause blindness and even death, says a report today . . . Babies infected at birth are likely to die or suffer serious handicap, says the report which launches a herpes education campaign. Once the virus has attacked, cold sores recur for life. In some cases sufferers can pass on the virus even when they do not have an active cold sore.

The article quoted the case of a father passing HSV to each of his children in turn as babies, who then needed hospitalisation, while their mother, who presumably had never before been in contact with HSV, became infected through breast-feeding her baby. This was an unusual and unfortunate case: had the mother been infected with HSV previously, in common with most of the adult population, she would have had antibodies and passed them to her babies *in utero*, so that their response to contact with their father's cold sores would have been far less serious.

A few months' later (February 1992) the magazine *Health and Fitness* carried an article by Jon Menon with the title 'Not So Simplex: time was, genital herpes was herpes and cold sores were just unsightly. Now doctors are reporting cross-infection' presenting herpes simplex as an ever-present threat:

Cold sores are contagious. Usually appearing around the mouth and nose, they can spread to other parts of the body and to other people through touching, kissing, oral sex, and sharing cups, cutlery and towels . . . in effect anybody can pass it on to anyone, anywhere at any age, from mouth to hands, mouth to genitals, hands to eyes.

The same article acknowledged that, according to experts, at least:

80% of the population are carriers of HSV, most picking up the virus in childhood or adolescence. The majority of people are symptomless.

The logic of this prevalence estimate is that the infection is endemic, that there is only 20 per cent of the population left to infect and that it is mostly harmless, and thus not a real threat. Acknowledged authorities on HSV had by that time been quoted in the press confirming that the virus is not passed on via cups, eating utensils and towels, etc. (Mindel and Carney 1991: 9). The Cold Sore Health Education Campaign was named at the end of the article for further information with the telephone number of the Rowland Company, a public relations company acting for Wellcome. This campaign was the subject of two complaints to the Prescription Medicines Code of Practice Authority which ruled on Wellcome's breach of the code on advertising prescription medicine to the general public.

Various leaflets about facial symptoms of HSV were produced at this time. A leaflet produced by the Rowland Company with support from the Wellcome Foundation was headed 'Cold sores?' and carried a picture of a mouth pinned open with stick figures attacking the lips with several implements including an axe. Underneath the picture was the caption 'consult your doctor or dentist'. Why people were to consult a practitioner was not made clear and if the millions of people who get facial symptoms of HSV occasionally, were to do so en masse there would be much wasted practitioner time. The impression both from the picture and the caption was somewhat alarmist. A more practical instruction might have been to consult a pharmacist. Included in a list of 'Do's and don'ts' was the injunction 'Do not kiss people, especially children'; and under the heading 'As extra precautions':

Do not share your eating and drinking utensils . . . the same towels or flannels with partners or family.

Another leaflet was produced with Boots' (the chemist) endorsement advertising Zovirax as a cold sore cream, 'a major breakthrough' and 'a unique new product recently introduced' (although Zovirax ointment had been prescribed for ten years by this time), claiming:

Now for the first time, if you treat the tingle you can prevent the cold sore appearing.

What was new was that Zovirax was now available over the pharmacist's counter without a prescription. The same injunctions as above were listed on this leaflet. At the end of the leaflet, there was an invitation to contact the Cold Sore Information Centre for more information. This leaflet acknowledged that most of the population carry the virus, and suggested that:

over 12 million people . . . get repeated attacks (around 1 in 5 of the population). They can have between 2 and 10 attacks a year.

In response to this campaign, the HA produced its own *Cold Sores* leaflet. The biggest difference between this leaflet and the others mentioned above, is in the tone and the list of 'do's and don'ts'. The HA pamphlet suggested use of a facial/lip sun block for those people whose recurrent symptoms are triggered by sunlight, and that discomfort caused by a 'cold sore' could be treated with an ointment or gel containing the anaesthetic lignocaine available without prescription. It commented that it is hard to avoid contracting HSV infection because it is so common and that, like other childhood infections, it is best caught when young (though not in babyhood) because this reduces the possibility of the very rare complications. The leaflet reassured that 'cold sores are rarely a cause for serious concern', and that 'most people who carry the virus do not experience recurrent symptoms'. It reminded its readers that 'cold sores are passed on from person to person via skin to skin contact' and will be infectious to people who have not previously come into contact with the virus, and that in such a case it could be passed to 'any part of another person's body by kissing'. The leaflet also pointed out that the infection may sometimes be transmitted when no symptoms are obvious.

The culmination of this ideological battle was a press briefing held at the Royal Society of Medicine in London on 16 June 1993 by the Herpes Association. This was presaged by an article in *The Times* by Jeremy Laurance on 10 June 1993 announcing that the association was about to publish a report 'showing how misrepresentation of the effects of herpes has increased the suffering of those affected by it'. The article also suggested that 'for some sufferers the social stigma is worse than the disease'. Although 'herpes was toppled from its perch as the most highly publicised sexually transmitted disease by Aids in the mid-1980s' and dating agencies for people with HSV had gone out of business, 'for sufferers . . . the stigma remains':

> though cold sores on the face and lips are caused by the same class of virus as those on the genitals, one is regarded as an uncomfortable affliction while the other is seen as a sign of moral turpitude.

At the press briefing, the Herpes Association launched their booklet *Herpes Simplex. A Guide* as 'a new independent information booklet . . . endorsed by the Society of Health Advisers (GU Medicine)' and presented a report with the title 'The Incidence of Herpes Simplex – Where is the Epidemic?'. There were presentations also from Dr David Barlow, GUM consultant from St

Thomas's hospital, Dr Gouri Dillon, a GP and medical journalist, and from three association members about their personal experiences. Dr Barlow went point by point through aspects of the condition which had been subject to misinformation. He reiterated the current medical consensus that it is transmitted by skin-to-skin contact and not via towels, and that it is extremely common, quoting a seroprevalence study which estimated that 90 per cent of the population were already infected with the virus by the age of twenty-five years. He suggested that most people were infected 'unknowingly', that during the primary episode of symptoms the condition was probably very infectious and that if people contracted HSV first in adulthood it 'can be a nasty affair' as 'any first attack of a virus in adulthood can be bad'. If the first attack was in the last two or three weeks of a pregnancy it had serious consequences, but where the woman had recurrent symptoms of HSV, the chances of passing it on (to the baby) were 'virtually nix'. He added:

> Of all the conditions I see in the GU clinic, the one that I have to spend longest talking to my patients about, is herpes. What they've been told is so awful and so frightening for them.

From Dr Gillon there was a plea to the press to 'set the record straight' and in one of the personal presentations a further impassioned plea:

> The frustration of listening to well over 300 callers, some of them extremely disturbed and distressed because they and society at large are not adequately informed, has given me the heart and strength to stand up and plead with you to please help educate those who are misinformed . . . to eradicate the terrible fear and cause and effect of the stigma attached to herpes simplex on the genitals, once and for all!

A cultural analysis of the role of the press will acknowledge that besides informing the public, the press also reflects and responds, and through the 'bandwagon effect', may produce a 'hype' around an issue. A news story may have a life of its own in the sense that it is a social phenomenon whose existence depends not only on press coverage, but also on those elements which make it 'newsworthy' and which reflect the culture and mores of the society from which it emerges; and it is the interaction between the press and these elements which provide the dynamic for a story to stay in the news.

The executive officer of the Herpes Association (Mike Wolfe) introduced his presentation questioning the claim of an epidemic of herpes simplex cases, by the following comments on the 'profoundly negative image of HSV' with its resultant detrimental effect on self image and loss of self-esteem:

> It is vital and indeed should be every individual's right to have accurate and factual information. It is wholly wrong to encourage people to feel worse than they need to. This benefits no-one other than those with vested interest . . . Symptoms of HSV, in the physical sense, will heal with or without treatment. For the vast majority it is the psychological aspect which is the greatest problem. It is the psychological trauma that we the HA deal with. This is a direct result of a manufactured hype.

Mr Wolfe presented an analysis of the 'hype of the eighties' which had resulted in:

> a profoundly negative perception of HSV, caused by the sensa-tional, inflammatory presentation on this subject. A great deal of misinformation caused fear and anxiety out of all proportion to the physical condition.

Although the press and media were being blamed for this, they had been given misleading information, he suggested. Furthermore, the hype had caused a conditioned response to the word 'herpes'. The terminology used to describe the condition such as 'incurable', 'disease', 'sufferers' and 'attacks' was 'descriptively inaccurate . . . profoundly negative . . . [and] wholly unhelpful to the individual', and, as many doctors agreed, 'inadequate'. It came from a time when there was a lack of understanding of the latency of the herpes viruses. Beyond this, the condition had been presented in terms of a worst-case scenario and theoretical possibilities, which was 'inap-propriate and damaging' and like a doctor telling a patient 'I'm sorry you have flu, X per cent of flu cases are fatal'.

Mr Wolfe's presentation went on to compare the incidence of cases of genital warts caused by the human papilloma virus (HPV) attending STD clinics during the 1980s with the incidence of HSV. Whereas all cases (recurrent and new) of HPV reached 77,000 by the end of the decade, the equivalent figure for HSV was no more than 19,000. He pointed out that this indicated a far more dramatic increase in genital warts than in genital symptoms of herpes simplex, that this was medically significant because of the established link between certain strains of HPV (3, 16, 18 and 33) and the development in women of cervical cancer and its precursors. He asked why so much attention had been given to herpes simplex when there were 'other more serious conditions like HPV'. His presentation also argued that the figures for cases of HPV in GUM clinics during the decade were inflated by people who were making repeat visits because of recurrences, some of them to seek the recently introduced treatment (acyclovir), and some of them visiting more than one clinic, and by an increasing proportion of women attending clinics rather than their GP. This argument was in line with a commentary accompanying the Communicable Disease Surveillance Centre data for the 1980s (Catchpole 1992).

The presentations were accompanied by a number of handouts including the new HA booklet and a forthcoming article in the association's newsletter summing up the evidence about acyclovir (Zovirax) based on the review in the *Drug and Therapeutics Bulletin* (Anon 1993), which concluded that the drug should be limited to those conditions where it is of proven value, namely in the treatment of a primary genital occurrence of HSV, ocular herpes simplex, herpes zoster (shingles) affecting the eye and as suppressive therapy for people with frequent genital symptoms. In other words, it was not recommended for the treatment of facial symptoms, nor for the treatment of episodes of recurrent genital symptoms, because it had been found to be relatively ineffective and was expensive. The association's attitude to acyclovir expressed in the executive officer's presentation was that:

> current medications are not the answer. At best they are useful to treat specific cases, e.g. primary symptoms . . . we believe that its development is not coincidental in relation to HSV becoming such an *important* issue.

Shortly after the HA press briefing, the *Sunday Times* (20 June 1993) carried an article by Neville Hodgkinson headed 'Drug firm accused of herpes scare tactics'. It began:

> A charity that seeks to improve understanding and treatment of herpes, the common virus infection, has accused a giant pharmaceutical company of scaremongering in a drive to promote the only drug licensed for use against the virus.

The article explained the HA's objections to literature distributed by Wellcome which it felt perpetuated a negative image of the condition, and continued:

> The arrival of AIDS put herpes in the shade for a while, and the Association felt a more realistic picture of herpes was beginning to be established . . . now . . . the company has launched a 'Wellcome Patient Care Initiative' targeting genital herpes, which it says can have 'a devastating effect on people's lives, causing deep and lasting damage to relationships'. The Association, and doctors supporting it, say that Wellcome's approach is contributing to the condition the drug is supposed to treat.

The article ended with an account of Wellcome's rejection of the criticisms in which a spokesperson had argued that 'in its anxiety to de-stigmatise herpes the Association was not giving sufficient weight to cases in which suffering does occur', and that:

> There is a significant minority of patients who seek advice and treatment. It is important that patients are made aware that the condition can be treated, certainly for someone suffering recurrent attacks of genital herpes . . . and about 2.5m people seek advice and treatment for (cold sores) from a pharmacist every year.

At the centre of the ideological battle which has raged over this common self-limiting viral condition, the main armies are in two opposing camps. The positions they have tended to take up have different implications and problematic aspects. One position is that herpes simplex is an extremely common condition which causes most people who have it no trouble. As people are very likely to come in contact with it sooner or later in their lives, it is better if they get it (HSV-1) sooner, when they are children because they are less likely to suffer serious symptoms or complications then, and will develop antibodies. If it causes recurrent symptoms, these will clear up by themselves without medical intervention. If you get recurrent symptoms in the genital area (likely to be HSV-2), this may be a nuisance, but need not prevent you having a fulfilling relationship and sex life, and you need not pass the infection to others. The motive behind this presentation is to reduce the highly negative and stigmatised image, and thus the psychosocial impact of the condition and the consequent suffering caused. The other position is that this is a condition which should be taken seriously because it is highly contagious, can cause serious problems and can be spread elsewhere – in particular, to the genitalia, to the eyes and to a newborn baby. However, there is a medical treatment available to provide relief from this dreadful condition. The motive behind this presentation is to get people to take sufficient notice of it to think they *ought* to do something about it, and to make sure that people seeking medical treatment know what is available. Overstating the position that herpes simplex is not nearly as dreadful a condition as it has been portrayed, carries with it the possible corollary that people suffering from its symptoms and asking for relief, will be viewed as not really needing scarce medical resources, nor deserving sympathy and understanding. Overstating the other position carries with it the danger of adding to the possibility of suffering for the vast majority of those experiencing the symptoms of the condition, by changing their conception of it to a more anxiety-provoking one.

The representation of herpes simplex is a story of how a hidden, intermittent, self-limiting condition ('genital herpes') became stigmatised, and a very common, accepted, and also minor, condition ('cold sores') became dangerous. It illustrates how a condition's portrayal in the public domain can make all the difference to people's thinking about it – and thus experience of it – over and above and their experience of physical symptoms.

Chapter 7

Conclusion
The significance of herpes simplex

This chapter will review the significance of herpes simplex as a condition in comparison with other conditions with which it has various similarities, and as a public health problem. It will also examine the way in which herpes simplex as a health problem illustrates the biopsychosocial matrix, its potential to affect a person's sense of self (identity) through its socially stigmatised meaning, its place in recent developments in virology and its reflection of new understandings in psychoneuroimmunology.

HSV SYMPTOM RECURRENCES IN COMPARISON WITH OTHER CHRONIC CONDITIONS

Like many other conditions which the current state of medical science cannot eradicate, and are thus chronic conditions, the symptoms of HSV infection are very variable and are largely unpredictable; however, they can be completely suppressed in many cases (with acyclovir or another antiviral agent), or ameliorated (with topical applications). HSV symptom recurrences along, with other chronic conditions, constitute an impairment which can become a handicap under certain circumstances. Where symptoms are 'cold sores' on the lips or face, the impairment/handicap is aesthetic rather than functional, easily visible, but not stigmatised. Where symptoms occur in the genital area, the impairment/handicap is psychosexual and, for the most part, invisible, but highly stigmatised. Whether the condition is experienced as a handicap of any sort depends on perceptions related to psychosocial aspects of the condition rather than its physical nature. The most significant difference between recurrences of HSV symptoms and other conditions normally thought of as chronic, is the fact that symptoms of

HSV infection reduce in severity and, usually, in frequency over a varying period of time – the condition gets better rather than worse. As with other chronic conditions produced by a virus such as HIV and hepatitis A, B or C, herpes simplex is infectious, though in a different way from HIV and hepatitis. It is only transmissible when the virus is being shed from the body's surface (skin or mucous membrane), where symptoms usually occur, during a reactivation of the virus. The rest of the time, the virus is inactive, and the condition cannot be passed on to another person. For the infection to be passed on, there must be skin-to-skin contact with the site of infection. HIV and hepatitis may be transmissible via body fluids at any time, though these conditions are more infectious at some stages than at others. Furthermore, HIV and hepatitis A, B or C have serious implications for an individual's future health status, while HSV, by itself, does not. The norm for recurrent symptoms of HSV infection is localised, self-limiting eruptions on the skin. Medical intervention is only required by an unlucky few who suffer particularly severe or frequent outbreaks of symptoms. In most cases, HIV infection gradually undermines bodily immunity leading to AIDS, and hepatitis – though it may remain latent for many years – has the potential to damage vital organs, so that medical intervention is needed with these viral conditions in order to try to preserve the individual's health as long a possible. HSV infection, like cytomegalo-virus (CMV) infection, is endemic rather than confined to a minority of the population, as HIV and hepatitis currently are in developed countries.

There are parallels between herpes simplex recurrences and other skin conditions, since symptoms occur on the skin and may be visible. The effect of severe psoriasis on the quality of life of patients attending outpatient clinics throughout the UK was investigated using self-complete questionnaires containing the Psoriasis Disability Index (PDI) (Finlay and Coles 1995). The questions were designed to assess the value placed by patients on the effects of their disease, using utility techniques of comparison with financial and time parameters, and with other diseases. The aim of the survey was to quantify the level of handicap experienced by patients with severe psoriasis and to assess the value they placed on their disease. The mean age of participants was forty-seven years and the mean time the patients had suffered from psoriasis was nineteen years. The survey 'confirmed the clinical impression that patients with severe psoriasis suffer significant disability, which results in considerable handicap' and that 'all aspects of their lives may be affected by their skin disease' (Finlay and Coles 1995). Of the 46 per cent of the sample currently working, 59 per cent said that they had lost time off work because of their psoriasis during the preceding year; and of those not working or retired, a third attributed their not working to their psoriasis. Nearly half of the sample stated that they would be prepared to spend two or three hours a day on treatment if this might result in normal skin the rest of the day. All except five of the 369 participants said they would prefer to have a complete cure of their psoriasis than be given £1,000; 71 per cent that they would be prepared to pay £1,000 or more and 38 per cent that they would pay £10,000 for a cure of their psoriasis. The amount a participant would be prepared to pay for a cure, was significantly correlated with their PDI score. It seems likely that a similar attempt to assess the value to a person of *not* having HSV recurrences (or even not being infected with HSV at all), would demonstrate that people would be prepared to pay a very considerable amount immediately after diagnosis and this would reduce to very much less ten years later.

The condition is most likely to have its greatest impact physically and psychologically in the initial stages after the primary episode and diagnosis. A number of research studies have looked at the impact of more frequent recurrences of HSV symptoms on the lives of people in the first few years after diagnosis, but, as noted in Chapter 5, little is known about the role of herpes simplex recurrences in the lives and health-related activity of people who continue to have recurrences over a long period such as a decade, and what effect, if any, the condition has on their quality of life. It would appear that many years of living with intermittent herpes simplex recurrences tend to reduce the significance of the condition to an occasional nuisance, and that the only sphere of life in which it may intrude significantly is the sexual. For a small proportion of people, and for a combination of individual and social reasons, this intrusion may amount to a handicap which may have wider effects in other aspects of their lives and on their self-concept.

Recurrent symptoms are a reminder that the condition has not gone away and thus its possible consequences, such as transmission of the infection to a sexual partner, are still a significant consideration. Whether recurrent symptoms cause distress tends to be determined as much if not more by their meaning to the individual at that point in his or her life, as by their physical characteristics (see review of individual cases in Chapter 5). As Fitzpatrick (1990: 47) underlines in his discussion of the social aspects of chronic illness:

> whilst symptoms have a strong coercive effect on the everyday life of the chronically sick, the personal meaning of symptoms may be of greater significance in determining the quality of life . . . many individuals may be relatively free from recurrent symptoms, but experience their illness as no less threatening, disruptive, or distressing.

Four episodes of 'mild to moderate' herpetic lesions per year might be viewed by one individual as of very little significance, as they get better without intervention and they interfere with her life hardly at all: she and her partner, who always uses a condom, do not have sexual intercourse for some days until they have healed. The same four episodes might be viewed by another person very differently. For this person, having the condition could be a determining factor in his approach to sexual relations, so that he is unwilling to risk rejection as a partner by disclosure to someone he cares for, and confines himself to occasional 'one night stands'; the symptom episodes remind him of what he perceives as his socially unacceptable secret and imply that his strategies to control their recurrence have failed. He often feels that his life is generally a failure and that he can never have a permanent and fulfilling partnership.

However, recurrent HSV symptoms, unlike the symptoms of many chronic conditions, do not interfere with the individual's capacity to carry out basic tasks of living, even if on occasion they result in some intermittent restriction of sexual activity. They may be inconvenient and unpleasant, but they will go away within a few days without any intervention and without significantly affecting the individual's overall health or health prospects. Nonetheless, many will not wait passively for the next visitation, but wish to be proactive and to try to have some control over recurrences. The range of elements which may be involved in an individual's prevention strategy were reviewed in Chapter 3 and tend to be an idiosyncratic mix of dietary alterations, stress reduction techniques, relaxation and rest prescriptions, complementary therapies, cognitive adjustments and medical intervention. The way in which control strategies might vary over time for a particular individual according to their circumstances was discussed in Chapter 5.

Like a persistent, unwelcome, intermittent visitor, recurrent recognised symptoms of herpes simplex oblige the individual to have some kind of relationship with it. This relationship may be one of acceptance and adjustment, or inharmonious, and will reflect the meaning the condition has for the individual at that point in their life. This meaning may or may not, in turn, reflect the socially constructed meaning, but is likely to be more idiosyncratic the longer a person has had the condition. So, for one informant with long-term recurrences of HSV symptoms, this condition was a spiritual lesson and an intermittent reminder of her imperfection as a human being/body; while for another, it was what was getting in the way of her being a full player in the game of life. Many view it is 'a monitor twitch on [their] state of well being' as one person expressed it – telling them that they are 'under the weather', 'run down', or have 'overdone it'. For many others, it simply has nuisance value and is nothing more than an occasional irritation. These meanings are a long way from the more dramatic and negative constructions which have been expressed by some individuals recently diagnosed, such as 'the end of my love life' or even, for a suicidal moment, 'the end of my life'. In the process of coming to terms and learning to coexist with the condition, accurate information undermining myths and worst case scenarios, and empathic support and acceptance, particularly from people with whom the individual identifies or who are important in his or her life, are important. Medical intervention in the form of suppressive therapy and psychosocial intervention in the form of support groups, or deliberately therapeutic groups, can help to encourage a positive adaptation in which the impact of the condition on the individual's life and identity is minimised.

HERPES SIMPLEX AND PERSONAL IDENTITY

Examination of the experiences of people with recurrences of HSV symptoms illustrates how:

> The relationship between self and identity in chronic illness is a social process which alters through time, as the bodily contingencies change.
>
> (Kelly and Field 1996)

A reduction in the frequency of symptoms (as with a favourable change in social circumstances) tends to lessen the influence of the condition on a person's self-identity. Writing about the implications for researchers of the findings of her study of people with chronic conditions, Charmaz (1987) also emphasised the need to look at people's experiences at different points in their illness trajectory in order to understand the processes of identity shifts and changes:

> The concept of identity levels promotes a search for changes in these levels and delineating the conditions under which they occur. It also promotes studying chronic illness over time and developing a clearer view of the ways that experiencing illness affects identity throughout the person's life.
>
> (Charmaz 1987)

Charmaz provided a framework for understanding the impact of chronic conditions on self and identity which can be applied to the experiences of people living with HSV symptom recurrences. The hierarchy of 'preferred' identity levels suggested by Charmaz reflected the 'relative difficulty of achieving specific aspirations and objectives' and ranged from the supernormal social identity, the restored self, the contingent personal identity to the salvaged self.

The 'restored self' is the identity level aimed for by individuals who anticipate the resumption of their former lives. They hope and believe they can return to being themselves again. Charmaz delineated different types of restored selves. The 'entrenched self' is an individual who simply wants to return to unchanged patterns of action, conviction and habit which had been built over the years and become a source of self-respect. The 'developing self' is a restored self with a commitment to growth and development in the future rather than to specific prior activities. The 'assumed self' is a self-concept situated in assumptions about significant social relationships and social worlds with which they have long been associated – often this identity is merged within an intimate relationship. A 'contingent personal identity' is one which is recognised as uncertain, but possible, and conditional on the illness or condition not intruding. Charmaz suggests that individuals who settle on this identity level require to translate the meanings of their condition into concrete problems to handle in relation to the intrusiveness of their symptoms or treatment, and this requires thought and some planning and organising. The identity level of the 'restored self' and the 'contingent personal identity' are the most relevant of Charmaz's concepts of identity levels to people diagnosed with HSV infection. Whether an individual identifies with the former rather than the latter, might well depend on whether they have or have had a sexual partner who accepts or accepted their condition.

For those individuals for whom recurrence of HSV symptoms is experienced as a significant handicap the 'salvaged self' may be the identity level they feel is appropriate to the circumstances of their condition. These individuals develop strategies to salvage positive self-images despite their reduced ability to function, but 'they hold little hope of realising typical adult identities in the outer world' (Charmaz 1987). If an individual diagnosed with HSV-2 infection believes (erroneously) that they will be unable to have a sexual relationship or to produce children 'normally' because of the infection, they are ruling out typical adult identities relating to sexual activity and procreation, and may be in the position of needing to rely on other activities in life, such as work, to sustain a positive self-image. If they allow the stigmatised image of 'herpes' to dominate their self-concept to an extent that renders them socially unacceptable in their own eyes, and dwell on their assumed loss of adult sexual and procreative functioning, they may have difficulty salvaging a 'self' at all. Charmaz observed that preoccupation with loss could inhibit the development of a 'salvaged self'.

In her discussion of the hierarchy of identity levels proposed by Charmaz, the assumption is that most people with chronic illness would aim for a higher identity level at first, but later settle for an identity lower in the hierarchy as they adjusted their hopes and plans to a deterioration in their condition or to their more realistic assessment of the limitations the condition imposes. She allowed, however, that:

A few, who initially were immersed in illness, moved up the identity hierarchy. For them salvaging a self was the first step.

(ibid.)

This kind of response is the more usual, as we have seen, for people diagnosed with HSV infection in the genital area. Those individuals who may at first feel devastated, and that their life has been ruined, may subsequently reassess the impact on their identity. Since the condition is not progressive and does not affect basic bodily or mental functions, it does not impose limitations in terms of work or usual social interaction; such individuals can feel therefore that there are many spheres of life unaffected by it in which they can feel affirmed and achieve their aims. Hopes for a long-term sexual relationship and parenthood, however, may feel rather more tentative and contingent on their negotiation of acceptance in a sexual relationship.

'The self is embedded in social relationships' as Charmaz expressed it, and thus personal and social identity tend to reflect each other, and the individual may incorporate socially-defined images of self within his or her definitions of personal identity. Charmaz uses the concept of identity to refer to attributes, actions and appraisals of self, reflecting past relationships and roles, as well as hopes, aspirations and future goals. The self-concept is thus an 'emergent structure' which may change 'as the person reflexively interprets the identifications and images that self and others confer upon him or her'. This explains why individuals with HSV-2 are vulnerable to the identification of having a socially unacceptable condition unless they can identify with other people who reject this image, or are presented with a non-stigmatised conception of the condition. Their acceptability as sexual partners may be disconfirmed or need negotiation:

> Responses to illness with their corresponding implied identity levels occur within social worlds and social relationships ... Others also define whether or not identity levels are 'appropriate', 'legitimate' and 'possible'. Preferred and potential identities become sources of *evaluation, negotiation, confirmation*, and *disconfirmation*.
>
> (Charmaz 1987)

Waxler's analysis of different social constructions of leprosy draws on a similar understanding of a socially-confirmed identity (Waxler 1981). There are a number of parallels between herpes simplex and leprosy in addition to the fact that they are conditions which appear on the skin. Both conditions are, or have been, highly stigmatised to an extent that people can feel the need for secrecy and social withdrawal. Both have been presented as incurable and highly contagious, and thus very threatening. Both conditions are, however, treatable and not life-threatening, and not even always communicable. Both herpes simplex and leprosy have been subject to attempted name changes as a way of dealing with the stigma associated with the names and redefining the condition. Leprosy was renamed Hansen's disease by the International Congress on Leprosy in 1948 and, as discussed in Chapter 4, the UK Herpes Association attempted to have herpes simplex referred to only as 'simplex' for a few years. A major difference between the two conditions is that leprosy may progress and cause physical malformations if untreated.

Waxler's argument is that:

> People diagnosed as having a particular disease learn 'how' to have it by negotiating with friends and relations as well as with people in the treatment system; this process is affected by society's beliefs and expectations for that disease . . . sustained by social and organisational forces that may have little to do with the disease itself as a biological process.

In relation to leprosy, she shows how the 'moral definition' of the condition varies between cultures and that there are different expectations in different societies – leprosy is not universally stigmatised – and thus people in one place discovering they have the disease will behave differently from the way they would in another. In India, the response to individuals with leprosy is repulsion and physical and social rejection, and a leper is likely to accept the stigma and exclude themselves from family and social life. Among the Hausa in Northern Nigeria, however, the disease has been very prevalent, but not been viewed with any special concern or disgust, so that people with leprosy have mostly lived a normal life with their families (Shiloh 1965).

It is the fact that the prevalence of HSV infection is hidden which allows a minority of the infected population to suffer a 'herpes'-associated stigma. The virus has existed successfully with its human hosts for at least a millennium. In the last decade and a half, however, its English-speaking human hosts have found it difficult to live knowingly with herpes simplex. The media presentation of the condition has been a crucial factor in this difficulty. Anne Karpf (1988: 143), in her analysis of media reporting of health and medicine in terms of 'moral panics' and 'miracle cures', suggests that:

> The herpes scare, like the look-after-yourself obsession, reflected the prevailing economic and social retrenchment. In the media, herpes (like food) was as much about the Lean and Moral Eighties as about physical illness. And remarkably, media coverage of a minor, at worst troublesome, condition was almost identical to that of a debilitating, and almost invariably killing one – AIDS.

The description of people's experiences in this volume has

demonstrated how living with recurring HSV symptoms involves managing both the physical symptoms and the social image of the condition. Coping with the social image of herpes simplex has required accurate and balanced information, support from others, identity maintenance work, as well as the courage to negotiate one's acceptability as a sexual partner. Some people with recurrent HSV symptoms have been fortunate: their symptoms are in an acceptable place on the body such as their lip; or they have received the information and support they needed to preserve their identities as socially acceptable persons; others have been less fortunate and have felt the need to be secretive and to hide themselves from the world.

THE SIGNIFICANCE OF HSV AS A PUBLIC HEALTH PROBLEM

Although HSV infection is endemic, the seroprevalence for HSV-1 or HSV-2 varies according to the population, as discussed in Chapter 1. Most people do not regularly have symptoms of the infection and the numbers presenting to GUM clinics in the UK for medical help are considerably lower than for HPV or chlamydial infections, which may have significant medical consequences in the genital tract, particularly for women. However, as a worldwide public health problem, HSV has significance because the symptoms include sores which carry the risk of further infection in unprotected sexual intercourse.

In a review of HSV infections during the decade since acyclovir was licensed, Corey (1993) suggests that:

> Perhaps the most significant development in the epidemiology of genital HSV-2 in the decade 1982–92, was the recognition of genital ulcer disease, and HSV infection in particular, as risk factors in the transmission and acquisition of HIV infection.

Two prospective studies have indicated that HSV-2 is often acquired prior to HIV-1 (Holmberg et al. 1988; Stamm et al. 1988). There is evidence, particularly from sub-Saharan Africa, that genital symptoms of HSV-2 infection are a possible risk factor for the acquisition of HIV-1 in heterosexual men and women. The suggestion is that the rapid transmission of HIV infection in this heterosexual population is due to the widespread prevalence of genital ulcer disease: chancroid, T. pallidum infection and HSV-2 (Corey 1993). A study carried out in a south London GUM clinic among fifty-one patients (thirty-five women and sixteen men, mostly African) who were HIV-seropositive and assumed to have acquired the disease through heterosexual transmission, investigated the cumulative incidence of sexually transmitted disease through a retrospective review of the case notes (O'Farrell and Tovey 1994). These investigators concluded that:

Although neither a cause nor effect relationship between genital herpes and HIV could be determined it is likely that both effects are operative, that is – genital herpes may both predispose to HIV acquisition and recur more often in HIV-positive individuals.

(O'Farrell and Tovey 1994)

Two studies, quoted by O'Farrell and Tovey, which examined the relationship between the numbers of recurrences of genital herpes and the degree of immunosuppression, came to different conclusions. Conflicting results have also been obtained in relation to genital herpes as a risk factor for HIV transmission in gay men. Whether it would be beneficial to counsel all GUM clinic patients with HSV-2 in relation to the risk of HIV transmission is, O'Farrell and Tovey (1994) suggest, unclear:

These individuals are at greater risk of acquiring HIV via heterosexual transmission but in low prevalence areas benefits from safer sex counselling must be weighed against increased anxiety in those already under stress from coming to terms with the possibility of recurrences of genital herpes.

The question would appear to be as much one of when and how to counsel in this respect, so as not to increase anxiety unnecessarily, than whether to do so at all. The UK Herpes Association guide, *Herpes Simplex*, both reassures and warns directly:

You are at no greater risk of contracting HIV than anyone else, as long as you avoid sexual contact when sores are present . . . if you have genital sores you should avoid genital contact as it could increase the risk from HIV infection.

The pamphlet explains that 'HIV infection and Herpes simplex are caused by totally different viruses which are NOT related', then goes on to explain why herpetic sores increase the risk of transmission because the 'lesions (breaks) in your skin makes it easier for HIV infection to enter your body'.

A problem of acyclovir-resistant virus has resulted from the increasing numbers of HIV-infected people in whom HSV may cause severe morbidity with atypical presentations who require prolonged suppressive antiviral regimens, and of iatrogenically immunocompromised people requiring prophylactic treatment after organ transplantation. However, alternative drugs to acyclovir have recently been developed with a greater degree of bioavailability which may overcome this problem. Nonetheless:

HSV infection remains a world-wide epidemiological problem, a problem that while amenable to some forms of therapy awaits prevention.

(Corey 1993)

HSV AND DEVELOPMENTS IN VIROLOGY

While it first appeared that the advent of AIDS and the funding of research into HIV had detracted from research concern and involvement with HSV, it now looks as if the management of HSV infection may well benefit from developments in modern virology that have resulted from attempts to deal with the worldwide threat of HIV infection and AIDS. Dr Michael Hall (head of the chemotherapy division of Roche Products) was quoted as telling a meeting of the British Association for the Advancement of Science that advances in genetic engineering had given greater insights into viral molecular biology that could not have been imagined ten years ago, with the result that anti-viral drug research had been catapulted to the top priority of many drug companies and research institutes around the world (*The Times*, 26 August 1987: 4).

Immunotherapy can work through non-specific stimulation of the immune system (by drugs such as isoprinosine (Immunovir) or administration of adjuvant preparations), or by direct stimulation of the immune system by vaccination. However, a study comparing the suppressive efficacy of Immunovir to acyclovir, demonstrated no clinical benefit for patients with HSV symptoms with the former drug (Kinghorn et al. 1992). There have been a number of attempts to develop a successful vaccine against HSV infection and many media reports of 'breakthroughs'. Gordon Skinner and his team of microbiologists at Birmingham Virus Research Unit developed and used one of these vaccines. Summarising the usefulness of these interventions in 1993, he wrote:

The history of attempts to modify the pattern of recurrent

herpetic disease by vaccination has been long, valiant but not unrewarding ... The totality of evidence – particularly from placebo-controlled studies during the last 10 years – suggests a measure of disease modulation by most vaccine formulations.

(Skinner 1993)

Another specialist in the treatment of HSV infections had a different view of these earlier vaccines:

Unfortunately there is no convincing scientific evidence that any of those thus far produced have any effect.

(Mindel and Carney 1991: 59)

Several different types of vaccines have been produced. The most recently developed type consists of intact or truncated glycoproteins produced by recombinant DNA technology. A vaccine developed by the Medical Research Council's virology unit in Glasgow has been in use since 1993 to boost the immune response of people troubled by recurrent genital symptoms of HSV. It appears that a live attenuated vaccine for Varicella-zoster Virus (VZV) can similarly boost the immunity of elderly individuals, and this may prevent or minimise herpes zoster outbreaks (Levin et al. 1992). Live attenuated (recombinant) purified glycoprotein, and recombinant-derived subunit HSV vaccines are currently being field-tested. The trials are investigating the potential for preventing primary infection, and for decreasing the frequency and severity of recurrences. Mindel (1996) reported a recent double-blind placebo-controlled trial of this vaccine in patients with frequently recurring genital symptoms of HSV infection which showed that vaccine recipients had significantly fewer recurrences and a marked and sustained increase in antibodies; however, they also experienced more episodes consisting of prodromal symptoms only, and this may suggest subclinical viral reactivation with a continuing risk of transmission. If the vaccination of people without immunity can protect them from acquiring HSV-2 infection, 'it will have a major impact on the incidence and morbidity of genital herpes' (Mindel 1996). In any consideration of the possibility of offering the vaccination to the general population, the cost factor will be uppermost, particularly since:

The majority of people exposed to herpes never develop any clinical problems, and in most of those who do the problems are minimal.

(Mindel and Carney 1991: 59)

If it proves successful, the vaccine is most likely to be offered to non-immune partners of individuals with HSV-2 infection.

Even the quality of the herpes virus which has proved problematic in the development of a vaccine to prevent infection – its ability to lie dormant in nerve cells – may be put to a good use in a development by a team of British virologists at University College London Medical School, which may result in a more effective and longer-lasting treatment for Parkinson's disease. The idea is that if the virus could be engineered to make dopamine it could act as a vector, carrying the genetic recipe for dopamine into the brain cells. The team is attempting to develop a safe way of doing this by specific modifications of the herpes virus.

HSV, PSYCHONEUROIMMUNOLOGY AND THE BODY

The majority of human bodies harbour the herpes simplex virus without people knowing it or being troubled by it. Recurrence of symptoms of this viral infection is a prototypical stress-associated condition. It takes advantage of its human host's vulnerability when the physiological system is under stress, whether that stress is because of illness, lack of sufficient rest or sleep, as a result of psychological distress, or some other factor. While most of the time the immune systems of the majority of the population infected with the virus prevent it from expressing itself symptomatically, a minority are regularly or intermittently troubled. The combination and balance of factors which keep the expression of the virus repressed in one person and not another is still a mystery. Various possible mediating factors such as self-esteem, cognitive coping mechanisms, locus of control and social support have been implicated in the association between biopsychosocial factors and HSV symptom recurrences. There is extensive evidence that lack of social support, life stress and depression are associated with one another, but the mechanism of their association is controversial (Vilhjalmsson 1993). Similarly, there is much evidence that social support and health are positively associated, but no significant correlations have so far been demonstrated between the measure of psychological or social support and *objective* measures of health status (Green 1993). According to Ader, Cohen and Felten (1995), concluding their discussion of developments in psychoneuroimmunology, there is a shift of understanding about the immunoregulatory function and 'a new appreciation of the interactions between behavioural, neural, endocrine and immune processes'. While there is also substantial evidence of a relationship between stress and decreases in both functional and enumerative measures of the immune system, including antibody titres to herpes viruses, it is currently unclear whether these changes have substantial implications for health (Herbert and Cohen 1993).

What is clear is that the herpes simplex virus is caught up in a complex matrix of factors at the heart of psychoneuroimmunology. A condition which is, for the most part, a common, self-limiting, minor skin condition, nonetheless exemplifies the complex interrelationships within different bodily systems and between the embodied person and the social context. The need for a biopsychosocial model of a health problem is amply demonstrated by the problem of HSV symptom recurrences. Description in purely biomedical terms does not begin to explain the nature of the degree of distress which has been associated with this condition. Including the psychological and the social dimensions allows for the attribution of both personal and cultural meaning to the condition, the mystery of its intermittent expression in the form of recurrent symptoms in some individuals, and the great range of different life experiences with herpes simplex.

References

Ader, R., Cohen, N. and Felten, D. (1995) 'Psychoneuroimmunology: interactions between the nervous system and the immune system', *Lancet* 345: 99–103.

Ades, A. E., Peckham, C. S., Dale, G. E., Best, J. M. and Jeansson, S. (1989) 'Prevalence of antibodies to herpes simplex virus types 1 and 2 in pregnant women, and estimated rates of infection', *Journal of Epidemiology and Community Health* 43: 53–60.

Adler, M. W. and Mindel, A. (1983) 'Genital herpes: hype or hope?' (editorial), *British Medical Journal* 286: 1767–8.

American College of Obstetricians and Gynecologists (ACOG) (1988) 'Perinatal herpes simplex virus infections', *ACOG technical bulletin* No. 122, Washington DC: American College of Obstetricians and Gynaecologists.

Anon (1992) 'Acyclovir in General Practice', *Drug and Therapeutics Bulletin* 30(26): 101–4.

Bassett, I., Donovan, B., Bodsworth, N. J., et al. (1994) 'Herpes simplex virus type 2 infection of heterosexual men attending a sexual health centre', *Medical Journal of Australia* 160: 697–700.

Beardsley, J. (1993) 'Education to undermine a taboo. Understanding herpes simplex virus', *Professional Nurse* 8(5): 322–6.

Blank, H. and Brody, M. (1950) 'Recurrent herpes simplex: a psychiatric and laboratory study', *Psychosomatic Medicine* 12: 254–60.

Bowman, C. A., Woolley, P. D., Herman, S., Clarke, J. and Kinghorn, G. R. (1990) 'Asymptomatic herpes simplex virus shedding from the genital tract whilst on suppressive doses of oral acyclovir', *International Journal of STD and AIDS* 1: 174–7.

Breinig, M. K., Kingsley, L. A., Armstrong, J. A., Freeman, D. J. and Ho, M. (1990) 'Epidemiology of genital herpes in Pittsburgh: serological, sexual and racial correlates of apparent and inapparent herpes simplex infection', *Journal of Infectious Diseases* 162: 299–305.

Brookes, J. L., Haywood, S. and Green, J. (1993) 'Adjustment to the psychological and social sequelae of recurrent genital herpes simplex infection', *Genitourinary Medicine* 69: 384–7.

Brown, Z. A., Benedetti, J., Ashley, R., et al. (1991) 'Neonatal herpes simplex virus infection in relation to asymptomatic maternal infection at the time of labor', *New England Journal of Medicine* 324: 1247–52.

Burnette, M., Koehn, K., Kenyon-Jump, R., Hutton, K. and Stark, C. (1991) 'Control of herpes recurrences using progressive muscle relaxation', *Behavior Therapy* 22: 237–47.

Carmack, M. N. and Prober, C. G. (1993) 'Neonatal herpes: vexing dilemmas and reasons for hope', *Current Opinion in Pediatrics* 5: 21–8.

Carney, O., Ross, E., Bunker, C., Ikkos, G. and Mindel, A. (1993) 'The effect of suppressive oral acyclovir on the psychological morbidity associated with recurrent genital herpes', *Genitourinary Medicine* 69: 457–9.

—— (1994) 'A prospective study of the psychological impact on patients with a first episode of genital herpes', *Genitourinary Medicine* 70: 40–5.

Carver, C. S., Scheier, M. F. and Weintraub, J. K. (1989) 'Assessing coping strategies: a theoretically based approach', *Journal of Personality and Social Psychology* 56: 267–83.

Catchpole, M. A. (1992) 'Sexually transmitted diseases in England and Wales: 1981–1990', *Communicable Disease Report* 2 (Review No. 1): 1–7.

Catotti, D. N., Clarke, P. and Catoe, K. E. (1993) 'Herpes revisited: still a cause of concern', *Sexually Transmitted Diseases* 20(2): 77–9.

Charmaz, K. (1987) 'Struggling for a self: identity levels of the chronically ill', *Research in the Sociology of Health Care* 6: 283–321.

Christenson, B., Bottiger, M., Svennson, A. and Jeannsen, S. (1992) 'A 15 year surveillance study of antibodies to HSV-1 and 2 in a cohort of young girls', *Journal of Infectious Diseases* 25: 147–54.

Collee, J. (1994) 'Complex Simplex', *Observer Life* 27 March.

Corey, L. (1993) 'Herpes simplex virus infections during the decade since the licensure of acyclovir', *Journal of Medical Virology Supplement* 1: 7–12.

—— (1994) 'The current trend in genital herpes: progress in prevention', *Sexually Transmitted Diseases* 21 (Suppl. 2): 38–44.

Corey, L. and Spear, P. G. (1986) 'Infections with herpes simplex viruses', *New England Journal of Medicine* 314: 686–91, 749–57.

Cunningham, A. L., Lee F. K., Ho, D. W. T., et al. (1993) 'Herpes simplex virus type 2 antibody in patients attending antenatal or STD clinics', *Medical Journal of Australia* 158: 525–8.

Dayan, L. (1994) 'Public criticism of doctors and herpes' (letter), *New Zealand Medical Journal* 28 September 1994: 381–2.

Donovan, B. and Mindel, A. (1995) 'Are genital herpes and warts really disappearing problems' (letter), *Australian Journal of Public Health* 19(2): 216–17.

Drob, S., Loemer, M. and Lifshutz, H. (1985) 'Genital herpes: the psychological consequences', *British Journal of Medical Psychology* 58: 307–15.

Finlay, A. Y. and Coles, E. C. (1995) 'The effect of severe psoriasis on the quality of life of 369 patients', *British Journal of Dermatology* 132: 236–44.

Fitzpatrick, R. (1990) 'Social aspects of chronic illness', in J. Hasler and T.

Schofield (eds) *The Management of Chronic Disease*, Oxford: Oxford Medical Publications.

Frenkel, L. M., Garratty, E. M., Shen, J. P., et al. (1993) 'Clinical reactivation of herpes simplex virus type 2 infection in seropositive pregnant women with no history of genital herpes', *Annals of Internal Medicine* 118: 414–18.

Goffman, E. (1963) *Stigma: notes on the management of spoiled identity*, Englewood Cliffs, NJ: Prentice-Hall.

Goldberg, L. H., Kaufman, R. H., Kurtz, T. O., et al. (1993) 'Continuous five-year treatment of patients with frequently recurring genital herpes simplex virus infection with acyclovir', *Journal of Medical Virology Supplement* 1:45–50.

Goldmeier, D. and Johnson, A. (1982) 'Does psychiatric illness affect the recurrence rate of genital herpes?', *British Journal of Venereal Diseases* 58: 40–3.

Goldmeier, D., Johnson, A., Byrne, M. and Barton, S., (1988) 'Psychosocial implications of recurrent genital herpes simplex virus infection', *Genitourinary Medicine* 64: 327–30.

Green, G. (1993) 'Editorial review: social support and HIV', *Aids Care* 5(1): 87–99.

Herbert, T. B. and Cohen, S. (1993) 'Stress and immunity in humans: a meta-analytic review', *Psychosomatic Medicine* 55: 364–79.

Herpes Association (UK) (1993a) 'Herpes Simplex. A Guide', London: Herpes Association.

—— (1993b) Press briefing, 16 June 1993, London: Royal Society of Medicine.

Holmberg, S. B., Stewart, J. A., Gerger, A. R., Byers, R. H., Lee, F. V., O'Malley, P. M. and Nahmias, A. J. (1988) 'Prior HSV type 2 infection as a risk factor for HIV infection', *JAMA* 259: 1048–51.

Hook, E. W., Cannon, R. O., Nahmias, A. J., et al. (1992) 'Herpes simplex virus infection as a risk factor for human immunodeficiency virus infection in heterosexuals', *Journal of Infectious Diseases* 46: 209–11.

Hoon, E., Hoon, P., Rand, K., Johnson, J., Hall, N. and Edwards, N. (1991) 'A psycho-behavioural model of genital herpes recurrences', *Journal of Psychosomatic Research* 35:25–36.

Jadack, R., Keller, M. L. and Hyde, J. (1990) 'Genital herpes: gender comparisons and the disease experience', *Psychology of Women Quarterly* 14: 419–34.

Johnson, R. E., Nahmias, A. J., Magder, L. S., et al. (1989) 'A seroepidemiology survey of herpes simplex virus type 2 infection in the United States', *New England Journal of Medicine* 321: 8–12.

Karpf, A. (1988) *Doctoring the media: the reporting of health and medicine*, London: Routledge.

Keller, M. L., Jadack, R. A. and Mims, L. F. (1991) 'Perceived stressors and coping responses in persons with recurrent genital herpes', *Research in Nursing and Health* 14: 421–30.

Kelly, M. P. and Field, D. (1996) 'Medical sociology, chronic illness and the body', *Sociology of Health and Illness* 18(2): 241–57

Kemeny, M., Cohen, F., Zegans, L. and Conant, M. (1989) 'Psychological and immunological predictors of genital herpes recurrence', *Psychosomatic Medicine* 51: 195–208.

Kinghorn, G. R. (1992) 'Addressing the psychosocial needs of genital herpes sufferers' (letter), *Genitourinary Medicine* 68(6): 424.

Kinghorn , G. R., Woolley, P. D., Thin, R. N., De-Maubeuge, J., Foidart, J. M. and Engst, R. (1992) 'Acyclovir versus Isoprinosine (Immunivor) for suppression of recurrent genital herpes simplex infection', *Genitourinary Medicine* 68: 312–16.

Knox, S. R., Corey, L., Blough H. A. and Lerner, A. M. (1982) 'Historical findings in subjects from a high socioeconomic group who have genital infections with herpes simplex virus', *Sexually Transmitted Diseases* 9(1): 15–20.

Koelle, D. M., Benedetti, J., Langenberg, A. and Corey, L. (1992) 'Asymptomatic reactivation of herpes simplex virus in women after the first episode of genital herpes', *Annals of Internal Medicine* 116: 433–7.

Koutsky, L. A., Stevens, C. E., Holmes, K. K., et al. (1992) 'Underdiagnosis of genital herpes by current clinical and viral-isolation procedures', *New England Journal of Medicine* 326: 1533–9.

Kulhanjian, J. A., Soroush, V., Au, D. S., et al. (1992) 'Identification of women at unsuspected risk of primary infection with herpes simplex virus type 2 during pregnancy', *New England Journal of Medicine* 326: 916–20.

Lacroix, J. M. and Offutt, C. (1988) 'Type A and genital herpes', *Journal of Psychosomatic Research* 32(2): 207–11.

Langenberg, A., Benedetti, J., Jenkins, J., et al. (1989) 'Development of clinically recognizable genital lesions among women previously identified as having asymptomatic herpes simplex virus type 2 infection', *Annals of Internal Medicine* 110: 882–7.

Levenson, J. L., Hamer, R. M., Myers, T., Hart, R. P. and Kaplowitz, L. G. (1987) 'Psychological factors predict symptoms of severe recurrent genital herpes infection', *Journal of Psychosomatic Research* 31(2): 153–9.

Levin, M. J., Murray, M., Rotbart, H. A., Zerbe, G. O., White, C. J. and Hayward, A. R. (1992) 'The immune response of elderly individuals to a live attenuated varicella vaccine', *Journal of Infectious Disease* 166: 253–9.

Longo, D. and Clum G. (1989) 'Psychosocial factors affecting genital herpes recurrences: linear vs mediating models', *Journal of Psychosomatic Research* 33: 161–6.

Longo, D. and Koehn, K. (1993) 'Psychosocial factors and recurrent genital herpes: a review of prediction and psychiatric treatment studies', *International Journal of Psychiatry in Medicine* 23(2): 99–117.

Longo, D., Clum, G. and Yaeger, N. (1988) 'Psychosocial treatment for recurrent genital herpes', *Journal of Consulting and Clinical Psychology* 56: 61–6.

Luby, E. D. and Gillespie, O. (1981) 'Psychological responses to genital herpes', *The Helper* 3(4): 2–3.

Luby, E. D. and Klinge, V. (1985) 'Genital herpes. A pervasive psychosocial disorder', *Archives of Dermatology* 121: 494–7.

McLarnon, L. and Kaloupek, D. (1988) 'Psychological investigation of genital herpes recurrence: prospective assessment and cognitive-behavioural intervention for a chronic physical disorder', *Health Psychology* 7: 231–49.

Manne, S. and Sandler, I. (1984) 'Coping and adjustment to genital herpes', *Journal of Behavioural Medicine* 7(4): 391–410.

Mertz, G. J. (1993) 'Epidemiology of genital herpes infections', *Sexually Transmitted Diseases in the AIDS Era* 7(4): 825–39.

Mertz, G. J., Benedetti, J., Ashley, R., et al. (1992) 'Risk factors for the sexual transmission of genital herpes', *Annals of Internal Medicine* 116: 197–202.

Mindel, A. (1990) 'Reluctance to prescribe suppressive oral acyclovir for recurrent genital herpes' (letter), *Lancet* 335: 1107.

—— (1993) 'Long-term clinical and psychological management of genital herpes', *Journal of Medical Virology Supplement* 1: 39–44.

—— (1996) 'Treatment and prevention of genital herpes', *Current Therapeutics* May 1996: 75–9.

Mindel, A. and Carney, O. (1991) *Herpes: what it is and how to cope*, London: Macdonald Optima.

Mindel, A., Faherty, A., Carney, O., et al. (1988) 'Dosage and safety of long-term suppressive acyclovir therapy for recurrent genital herpes', *Lancet* i: 926–8.

O'Farrell, N. and Tovey, S. J. (1994) 'High cumulative incidence of genital herpes amongst HIV-1 seropositive heterosexuals in south London', *International Journal of STD and AIDS* 5: 415–18.

Office of Population Censuses and Surveys (1992) *Communicable Disease Statistics* Series MB2, London: HMSO.

Patel, R., Cowan, F. and Barton, S. (1997) 'Advising patients with genital herpes' (editorial), *British Medical Journal* 314: 85–6.

Posner, T. (1990) 'H.A. membership survey follow up', *Sphere* (Journal of Herpes Association) 6(1): 1, 4–5.

Public Health Laboratory Service (1986) PHLS *Communicable Disease Report, Annual Tabulations.*

Rand, K., Hoon, E., Massey, J. and Johnson, J. (1990) 'Daily stress and recurrence of genital herpes simplex', *Archives of Internal Medicine* 150: 1889–93.

Roberts, S. W., Cox, S. M., Dax, J., Wendel, G. D. and Leveno, K. J. (1995) 'Genital herpes during pregnancy: no lesions, no cesarean', *Obstetrics and Gynaecology* 85(2): 261–4.

Robinson, I. (1988) *Multiple sclerosis*, London: Routledge.

Scambler, G. (1984) 'Perceiving and coping with stigmatizing illness' in R. Fitzpatrick et al. (eds) *The Experience of Illness*, London: Tavistock.

Schneider, J. and Conrad, P. (1981) 'Medical and sociological typologies: the case of epilepsy', *Social Science and Medicine* 15: 211–19.

Schur, E. (1979) *Interpreting deviance: a sociological introduction*, New York: Harper and Row.

Shiloh, A. (1965) 'A case study of disease and culture in action: leprosy among the Hausa of northern Nigeria', *Human Organization* 24: 140–7.

Siegel, D., Golden, E., Washington, A. E., et al. (1992) 'Prevalence and correlates of herpes simplex infections: the population-based AIDS in multiethnic neighborhoods study', *JAMA* 268: 1702–8.

Silver, P. S., Auerbach, S. M., Vishniavsky, N. and Kaplowitz, L. G. 'Psychological factors in recurrent genital herpes infection: stress, coping style, social support, emotional dysfunction, and symptom recurrence', *Journal of Psychosomatic Research* 30(2): 163–71.

Skinner, G. R. B. (1993) 'Chemotherapeutic and immunotherapeutic management of herpes genitalis', *Current Obstetrics and Gynaecology* 3: 225–31.

Slomka, M. J. (1996) 'Seroepidemiology and control of genital herpes: the value of type specific antibodies to herpes simplex virus' *Communicable Disease Report* 6; Review No 3: 41–5.

Spangler, J. G., Kirk, J. K. and Knudson, M. P. (1994) 'Uses and safety of acyclovir in pregnancy', *Journal of Family Practice* 38(2): 186–91.

Stamm, W. E., Handsfield, H. H., Rompalo, A. M., Ashley, R. L., Roberts, P. L. and Corey, L. (1988) 'The association between genital ulcer disease and acquisition of HIV infection in homosexual men', *JAMA* 260: 1429–33.

Stone, K. M., Brooks, C. A., Guinan, M. E. and Alexander, E. R. (1989) 'National surveillance for neonatal herpes simplex virus infection', *Sexually Transmitted Diseases* 16: 152–6.

Stout, C. and Bloom, L. (1986) 'Genital herpes and personality', *Journal of Human Stress* 12: 119–24.

Straus, S. E., Seidlin, M., Takiff, H., et al. (1989) 'Effect of oral acyclovir treatment on symptomatic and asymptomatic virus shedding in recurrent genital herpes', *Sexually Transmitted Diseases* 16(2): 107–13.

Strauss, A. L. (1975) *Chronic illness and the quality of life*, Saint Louis MO: C.V. Mosby Company.

Stronks, D. L., Rijpma, S. E., Passchier, J., Verhage, F., Van der Meijden, W. and Stolz, E. (1993) 'Psychological consequences of genital herpes, an explanatory study with a gonorrhea control-group', *Psychological Reports* 73: 395–400.

Swanson, J. M. and Chenitz, W. C. (1993) 'Regaining a valued self: the process of adaptation to living with genital herpes', *Qualitative Health Research* 3(3): 270–97.

Tilson, H. H., Engle, C. R. and Andrews, E. B. (1993) 'Safety of acyclovir: a summary of the first 10 years experience', *Journal of Medical Virology Supplement* 1: 67–73.

VanderPlate, C. and Kerrick, G. (1985) 'Stress reduction treatment of severe recurrent genital herpes virus', *Biofeedback and Self Regulation* 10: 181–8.

VanderPlate, C., Aral, S. and Magder, L. (1988) 'The relationship among genital herpes simplex virus, stress, and social support', *Health Psychology* 7: 159–68.

Vilhjalmsson, R. (1993) 'Life stress, social support and clinical depression: a reanalysis of the literature', *Social Science and Medicine* 37(3): 331–42.

Wald, A., Zeh, J., Barnum, G., Davis, L. G. and Corey, L. (1996) 'Suppression of subclinical shedding of herpes simplex virus type 2 with acyclovir', *Annals of Internal Medicine* 124: 8–15.

Wald, A., Zeh, J., Selke, S., Ashley, R. L. and Corey, L. (1995) 'Virological characteristics of subclinical and symptomatic genital herpes infections', *New England Journal of Medicine* 333: 770–5.

Watson, D. (1983) 'The relationship of genital herpes and life stress as moderated by locus of control and social support', unpublished manuscript, Long Beach CA: University of Southern California.

Waxler, N. E. (1981) 'Learning to be a leper: a case study in the social construction of illness' in Mishler E. et al. (eds) *Social Contexts of Health, Illness and Patient Care*, New York: Cambridge University Press.

Wellcome Australia. 'Genital herpes: a facts book', Wellcome Australia Limited.

Whitley, R. J. (1993a) 'Neonatal herpes simplex virus infections', *Journal of Medical Virology Supplement* 1: 13–21.

—— (1993b) 'Antiviral therapy: the time has come', *Journal of Medical Virology Supplement* 1: 1.

Whitley, R. J. and Gnann, J. W. (1992) 'Acyclovir: a decade later', *New England Journal of Medicine* 327(11): 782–9.

World Health Organization (WHO) (1990) 'Sexually transmitted infections increasing . . . ', *WHO Features* No. 152, Geneva: WHO Office of Information.

Wood, P. (1980) 'The language of disablement: a glossary relating to disease and its consequences', *International Rehabilitation Medicine* 2: 86–92.

Index

coverage 4–6, 8–9, 107, 108, 109,
110; orogenital 11, 16, 21, 77, 85;
prevention of 21, 22, 78–80;
suppressive treatment and 27
treatment, medical 26–9, 54, 55,
57–60, 114; instructions for
58–9; prophylactic *see*
suppressive treatment; of
recurrences 26–7; side-effects 28,
58; topical 54, 58–9, 91; vaccine
29, 126–8; *see also* acyclovir
Treponema pallidum 124
trichomoniasis 11, 12, 20
Turow, Scott: *The Burden of Proof*
10

ulcers 17, 20, 124–6
University College, London 128
urination, difficulty with 22
USA 13–14, 15, 24–5, 40, 43, 81

vaccine 29, 126–8
valaciclovir (Valtrex) 28–9
VanderPlate, C. 56, 95
varicella zoster virus 4, 15, 127
vidarabine 28
Vilhjalmsson, R. 128
vitamins 54, 55, 63, 91, 92

Wald, A. 21, 27
warts, genital 11, 12, 65, 78, 111–12
Watson, D. 95
Waxler, N.E. 122, 123
Weintraub, J.K. 60
Wellcome 26; and Herpes
Association 112–13; promotion
methods 57, 105–6, 108, 112–13
Wellcome Australia 21
Western blot assay 13
Whitley, R.J. 23, 24, 25, 26, 28
Woddis, Carole 100
Wolfe, Mike 101, 104, 111–12
Woman 62–3
women 12–13, 14–15, 17, 21–2;
acyclovir treatment 58–9;
doctors' attitudes 59–60
Wood, P. 83
World Health Organization 11

X-ray therapy 91
xylocaine 27

Yaeger, N. 56

Zovirax *see* acyclovir